What's So Funny About®...Diabetes?

A Creative Approach to Coping with
Your Disease

By RN, Humor Expert &
Speaker Hall of Fame inductee
Karyn Buxman

With random commentary
from a diabetes patient
["So let's get on with it, already!"]

Cover design by Poole Advertising
573-221-3635 | www.PooleAdvertising.com

What's So Funny About . . .? Publishing
Karyn Buxman
858-603-3133 | www.KarynBuxman.com

Table of Contents

Foreword

By Lee S. Berk, DrPH, MPH, FACSM, CVJES. CLS

I have spent most of my career researching the psychoneuroimmunological connections between the positive emotions of humor and their influence on health. It has been a rich and rewarding journey. Following in the footsteps of Norman Cousins and his research funding, various public, health and medical care communities have begun to understand and embrace the power of therapeutic humor. Humor has shown supportive beneficial effects on a large number of the body's essential processes. What a gift this now presents for people who have chronic conditions—among them, diabetes.

In this book, author Karyn Buxman, RN shows people who have diabetes specifically how to use humor to enhance the beneficial coping aspects in their lifestyle. She is uniquely qualified to do so. As a nurse she has hands-on healthcare therapeutic experience; as a performing world-class humorist, she has addressed thousands of people over the last 25 years. Combine that with her knowledge and expertise of the reality of the mind-body connection through the medical science of psychoneuroimmunology, you now hold in your hands a book full of new and genuinely helpful practical tools and techniques that use positive emotions and humor for managing your diabetes lifestyle. And, by-the-way, you'll get a good laugh as you read through this insightful book. You will find that the laughter and insights will remain with you as you continue to practice the techniques Karyn illustrates.

Humor and laughter are powerful. They translate from your mind/brain to your body. They produce very real physiological changes. You can experience real, tangible benefits right now by using these unique tools—and you will even experience benefits from them simply by thinking about how much fun you're going to have laughing later. Read, learn, laugh! You'll be glad you did.

~ Lee S. Berk, DrPH, MPH, FACSM, CHES, CLS

Director Clinical Molecular Research Laboratory
     School of Allied Health Professions—
     Loma Linda University
Faculty of Graduate Studies
     Associate Professor—School of Allied
     Health Professions
Associate Research Professor Pathology and
     Human Anatomy—School of Medicine
     Loma Linda University

Acknowledgments & Dedications

Whats so funny about diabetes? This book was written for many people: The people who know the answer to that question and for those who have yet to discover it. These pages were written for anyone who's ever pricked a finger, snuck a cupcake, or had to say "No thank you" when they wanted to scream "Yes!"

This book was written for my fellow nurses and for my colleagues in the field of therapeutic humor. You folks rock each and every day! You inspire, illuminate, imagine and implement a better world every day. I am honored to be in your company.

A high-five to my colleagues, mentors and friends at the Association for Applied & Therapeutic Humor. We are making the world a better place one laugh at a time.

A huge thank you to my editor Cindy Potts, whose talent, tenacity, and twisted sense of humor have made this project a blast!

Cheers to Peter and all the regulars at The Pacific Bean—as this was definitely a caffeine-fueled project.

And of course, this book would not be here were it not for my mildly brilliant and oh-so-romantic husband, Greg Godek.

Introduction

A priest, a rabbi, and diabetic walk into a bar and the bartender says, "Hey—what *is* this? Some kind of *joke?*"

What's so funny about diabetes? Well, maybe *nothing.* Then again, maybe *everything.* Especially if you understand the premise that so much of our humor comes from pain and discomfort—maybe it's our own, maybe it's somebody else's.

> *"Tragedy is when I cut my finger.*
> *Comedy is when you walk into an open*
> *sewer and die."*
> ~ Mel Brooks

We're not usually laughing about having a good hair day, or a sexy figure, or having more money than Donald Trump (and he's definitely *not* having a good hair day. But I digress…). We're laughing about the things that make us *crazy.* And let's face it, if you're a diabetic, you've got more than your fair share of pain and discomfort.

When you're a diabetic, you need to arm yourself with all the tools that you possibly can to become the healthiest person that you can be. You need a large repertoire of skills. Humor isn't the be-all and end-all; it's not meant to *replace* your medical regime, but rather to be a *complement* to all of the efforts that you're already making.

You may be thinking to yourself, "But *I'm* not funny. Can you *teach* me to be funny?" Well, yes. I could teach you a short comedy bit that might serve you every few weeks. But it's not about *being* funny as much as it is about *seeing* funny. If you can "see funny," the "be funny" will fall into place by itself.

Odds are that you *already* have a sense of humor. Selecting this book means that chances are even better that it's a *good* sense of humor. But I can help improve and focus your humor skills to refine them to make them stronger and more effective, so that they serve you and your special needs.

And here's a bonus. When you start using humor proactively to deal with your diabetes, you're going to find that humor helps you in a lot of other areas in your life, as well. That's because humor has physiological benefits; psychological benefits; it's a social lubricant—it helps strengthen relationships and rapport; and the more you use it, the easier it becomes.

As a diabetic, you're in the company of a lot of

funny folks such as Jack Benny, Delta Burke, Nell Carter, Jackie Gleason, Jerry Lewis, Mae West, Mary Tyler Moore, and Carroll O'Connor, just to name a few. (Diabetes doesn't necessarily make you funny, but it sure didn't get in the way of the success of these guys and gals!)

So fasten your seatbelt, put your tray in the upright and locked position, and let's go!

Yours in laughter!
Karyn Buxman, RN, MSN, CSP, CPAE

o **RN:** Registered Nurse
o **MSN:** Masters Degree in Mental Health Nursing
o **CSP:** Certified Speaking Professional (an earned designation)
o **CPAE:** Council of Peers Award for Excellence, also known as The Speaker Hall of Fame (a bestowed professional honor)

*"If we took what we now know
about laughter and bottled it,
it would require FDA approval."*

~ Dr. Lee Berk, psychoneuroimmunologist

Chapter 1

What's NOT So Funny About Diabetes?

A recent report indicates that the number of people with diabetes around the world has skyrocketed over the last two decades from 30 million to 230 million. That's an increase of nearly 700 percent. Some estimates project that this number could grow over the next two decades to 350 million people!

America's problem with diabetes is especially acute. Currently one in ten Americans has diabetes. Experts project that by 2050, that number could reach one in three! We're in the center of a diabetes epidemic, and that's no joke.

Diabetes is a serious disease. Being diagnosed is life changing. It's overwhelming, even terrifying, to contemplate the new level of responsibility and worry that comes when the doctor says, "I have some news for you. You'd better sit down."

To put this book in its proper perspective, perhaps we should take just a moment to look at the serious side of diabetes. While there *is* humor be found in your condition, the truth is that having diabetes is no joke, and not taking your disease seriously can have some nasty—if not deadly—consequences.

Here's what can happen if your diabetes gets out of control:

o   **Eye problems:** Diabetes can damage blood vessels in the eyes, which may lead to cataracts, glaucoma, diabetic retinopathy, macular degeneration and blindness. *["I don't understand most of those phrases— but they don't sound good."]* — (That's the first of many commentaries and reactions by a diabetes patient who reviewed this book.)

o   **Hearing problems:** Diabetics are twice as likely to suffer hearing loss as non-diabetics. *["Huh?!?"]*

o **Heart and blood vessels:** Diabetes can cause vascular problems including an increased risk of heart attack, stroke, peripheral vascular disease, high blood pressure and high cholesterol. *["Definitely not good."]*

o **Skin Problems:** Diabetes can result in skin ulcers and sores that won't heal, leading to foot problems and even amputation of limbs. *["Ouch!"]*

o **Nerve damage:** Diabetes can result in pain or numbness and problems with feet, intestines, the heart, and other organs. *["As if I don't have enough problems already."]*

o **Kidney disease and kidney failure:** Diabetes is the most common cause of chronic kidney disease (CKD) and kidney failure, accounting for 44% of all new cases. *["Does this mean I'll have to go on kidney dialysis?"]*

o **Sexual dysfunction:** Diabetes can cause sexual difficulties in both men and women. Men may have difficulty attaining or maintaining an erection. Women may experience vaginal dryness, making sex painful, or can lead to the loss of sensation in the genital area making orgasm difficult or impossible to achieve. *["Now **this** item is definitely going to motivate me!"]*

o **Depression:** This is a common issue for many people with diabetes. While everyone experiences the blues sometimes, chronic, ongoing depression is a debilitating condition that can negatively impact every aspect of your life. *["Can't I just pop a handful of anti-depressants?"]*

o **Cancer:** A recent study found that adults with diabetes had a 10% increased risk of developing any type of cancer compared to those without the disease. *["Could this get any worse??"]*

o And if that weren't bad enough, **diabetes can even make us get older faster!** According to a recent study, diabetes may speed up the aging process in middle-aged adults. Diabetics between 51 and 70 years of age were twice as likely to develop age-related ailments—like cognitive impairment (Alzheimer's or dementia), falls, dizziness, bladder problems and vision problems—than those without the disease.

Okay, so having diabetes is not fun or humorous. I'm not trying to make light of this serious disease. But while diabetes *itself* is not funny, your experiences and your life *can* be funny.

The premise of this book—borne out by scientific research—is that humor has many practical benefits for diabetes patients.

So let's get going!

"Humor is power"
~ Karyn Buxman, RN

Chapter 2
What Humor Can Do For You

Now some good news! Scientists are finally proving what most people have known since Biblical times: "A merry heart doeth good like a medicine." (Proverbs 17:22) *["Amen!"]*

In medieval times it was thought that if the body's fluids (known as "umors") were in balance, one was of good temperament—or healthy. That's where the phrase "having a good sense of humor" came from. The umors were yellow bile, blood, lymph, and black bile. Blood sugar wasn't specifically mentioned, but it should have been. After all, having balanced blood sugar can certainly help one's mood.

Throughout the Middle Ages, the practice of medicine was more art than science, and the mysterious art stagnated for many centuries. The following is from a

Saturday Night Live skit, with comedian Steve Martin playing Theodoric of York, a doctor/barber:

> *"You know, medicine is not an exact science,*
> *but we are learning all the time.*
> *Why, just fifty years ago, they thought a disease*
> *like your daughter's*
> *was caused by demonic possession or witchcraft.*
> *But nowadays we know that Isabelle is suffering from an*
> *imbalance of bodily humors,*
> *perhaps caused by a toad or a small dwarf*
> *living in her stomach."*

We now know that umor or humor isn't a body fluid at all (although any nurse will tell you that the topic of body fluids can be hysterically funny material for staff-only stories…).

But believe-it-or-not, scholars still can't agree on a single, simple definition of just what humor really is! Some of the things they *do* agree upon include: Humor is a mindset, a perspective, and something that tends to make you laugh. I know that seems obvious to you and me; but a researcher who is trying to analyze the effects of humor in a scientific manner needs to know exactly what he or she is measuring.

My Masters thesis was on the relationship between humor, health, and communication. During my research I discovered that few "experts" could agree upon what humor really is. One great definition comes from my colleague, Dr. Joel Goodman, founder of The HUMORProject, who said, "Humor is a childlike perspective in an otherwise serious adult reality." I love the idea of looking at life through the eyes of a child—they have such a sense of fun and playfulness (which we seem to lose as we get older, more serious, more "professional"). A different perspective is the underpinning of all reframing, our ability to see funny, and ultimately our ability to just be happier. *["Hey, I LIKE that!"]*

Humor is definitely a bit of a paradox (not to be confused with a pair-of-ducks). *["That's a groaner!"]*

Humor can come from surprise. Humor can come from "derailment"—that sudden twist that makes a good joke work so well. Humor can come from pure delight (watch young children for example; older folks don't experience nearly as much pure delight in living and discovering the world around them). And, believe it or not, sometimes humor and laughter can come from pain and discomfort (see: banana peel; or Wiley Coyote dropping an anvil on his own head, in the

pursuit of the Road Runner; or most practical jokes).
How important is humor? Consider this:

*"It is encouraging to know that something
like laughter, which is cost-free and can be shared
and promoted by many,
has beneficial effects on the well-being of a chronic disease
that affects 24 million Americans."*
~ Sue McLaughlin, President of Health Care and
Education for the American Diabetes Association

There's been lots of serious research into what
makes us laugh—and what laughter does for us. These
studies come from part of a bigger field of research
called psychoneuroimmunology (psycho=mind;
neuro=nervous system; immunology=immune system) or sometimes referred to as the mind-body connection. Some experts throw in the endocrine system,
too: psychoneuroimmunoendocrinology (I think these
scientists are frustrated Scrabble players). I'll refer to
psychoneuroimmunology as PNI from here on out.

Here are the highlights of that research, particularly as it pertains to people with diabetes.

What Humor Can Do for Your *Body*

*"The old man laughed loud and joyously, shook up the
details of his anatomy
from head to foot, and ended by saying such a laugh was
money in a man's pocket, because it cut down
the doctor's bills like everything."*
~ Mark Twain

Humor and laughter have many positive effects on your body. We're really in the infancy of PNI, but early indications are that there are positive benefits for almost every body system: Cardiovascular, respiratory, immune, and musculo-skeletal just to name a few. But some of these effects are going to be of more interest to you than others.

*"While there is no reason to expect humor to be helpful in
preventing diabetes, it is helpful in managing it."*
~ Dr. Paul McGhee, author of
Humor: The Lighter Path to Resilience and Health

Let's Get to The Heart of The Matter

Humor can help people with diabetes reduce their cholesterol. In a study conducted by psychoneuroimmunologist Dr. Lee Berk, and his endocrinologist and diabetes specialist colleague, Dr. Stanley Tan, patients with Type 2 diabetes spent half an hour a day watching movies or sitcoms that they found humorous. As a result, their levels of HDL (the *good* cholesterol) increased by 26%, while harmful C-reactive proteins declined by 66%. When was the last time you heard that watching TV could actually make you healthier? *["Um, never!"]*

Reducing cholesterol is a great idea, as it reduces your risk for cardiovascular disease. Having diabetes increases your risk for cardiovascular disease up to four times, so we're still swimming upstream here. Reducing cholesterol is one example of how humor can do more than make you *feel* better: Humor can help you be *healthier!*

Laughter helps lower your blood pressure and increase circulation. Maintaining optimal circulation is absolutely critical. It's so important for you to keep the blood moving to the extremities, flowing to your fingers and toes. Circulation is important because a constant, fresh supply of oxygenated blood speeds healing and helps keep minor wounds from becoming major problems.

Blood Sugar (Blood Glucose) Control

Does your blood sugar spike after suppertime? Humor can help lower the increase in blood sugar you experience after eating a meal. A research study from Japan showed that those who watched a brief comedy show after eating had lower glucose values than those who did not see the program.

Over two days, participants were given identical meals. On one day, they watched a humorless lecture, and the next they watched a Japanese comedy show. The group of 19 people with diabetes and five without had their blood glucose monitored during the study.

While non-diabetics showed no difference in blood glucose following the serious lecture or the comedy show, diabetics showed significantly lower blood glucose levels following the comedy show, but not the boring lecture. (The study was published in

Diabetes Care.) The glucose reducing effect of humor was replicated in three additional studies. While the scientists can't yet put their finger on *exactly* what's responsible for the blood-glucose lowering effect in diabetics, the researchers suggest that these findings point to "the importance of daily opportunities for laughter in patients with diabetes." *["This is exciting news!"]*

Studies show that laughing lowers your levels of the stress hormones cortisol and adrenaline. Cortisol increases insulin resistance, while adrenaline tells your liver to pump more glucose into your blood. The combined effect can be a lasting reduction in blood glucose levels. In other words, laughter can probably help lower your blood glucose and keep it down for quite a while!

Microvascular Complications of Diabetes

High blood sugar levels stimulate an enzyme in your blood called renin. (Now hang in here with me while I get technical for a minute.) *["Is that a REAL minute or a NURSE'S minute?!"]* Renin helps produce a protein called angiotensin, which among other things, causes constriction of blood vessels. Individuals with diabetes have higher levels of renin in their blood and this increase in renin levels appears to be related to vascular complications, often in the kidneys, retina, or nervous system. (This is why diabetics suffer more than non-diabetics from chronic kidney disease [CKD], diabetic retinopathy and blindness, and numbness or pain in their extremities.)

The Japanese research team mentioned above conducted another study measuring levels of renin and angiotensin. This time they exposed diabetics and non-diabetics to a six-month regimen of watching comedy videos once a week. *["I want to meet these researchers—they sound like fun!"]* At the beginning of the study, the diabetics' levels of renin were five times higher than typical non-diabetics. Now here's the really interesting part: By the third month of the study, the renin levels of the diabetic patients dropped (and stayed down through the rest of the study), on average, by 2/3! This drop put half of the diabetic subjects into the normal range.

At the same time, angiotensin levels dropoped over the first three months of watching these humorous videos (and stayed down the remainder of the study). The researchers went as far to conclude that "laughter therapy can be used as a non-pharmacologic treatment for the prevention of diabetic microvascular complications."

It's In Your Genes

I would be remiss if I did not include this one last bit of information about new research on humor, laughter, and your genes (no, not your *jeans*—I'm talking about smaller than cellular level here). Lest your eyes glaze over from too much detail (but email me if you DO want more information about this)—let me try to summarize for you yet another study by our wonderful Japanese researchers (mentioned above).

Our team measured yet another enzyme, prorenin (a pre-cursor to renin, and involved in diabetic complications). This enzyme was increased in the diabetics participating in their study. Using their design as mentioned above (boring lecture versus comedy shows) the levels of prorenin dropped sharply after watching the comedy shows. AND the even bigger news: Laughter "normalized the expression of the prorenin receptor gene . . . this demonstrated the inhibitory effects of laughter on the onset/deterioration of diabetic complications at the gene-expression level."

Whew! Let me translate that into layman's terms. *["Please!"]* Humor and laughter may not just affect your health at the cellular level—which is already good news. It may affect your health positively at the genetic level which would affect you and those whom you pass your genes along to! Great news—and fodder for researchers to tackle in the years to come. *["Do these genes make me look fat?"]*

Pain Management

Pain management is part of every person with diabetes' life. Diabetes comes with its own unique set of aches and pains. From tender fingertips to overall fatigue, there's an element of pain management that's inherent in taking charge of your diabetes.

Laughter lowers blood pressure and reduces anxiety and inflammation. This helps relieve pain throughout the body (pain *outside* your body is beyond our scope of practice—sorry! Our humor seems to be of little help in fighting politics or global warming.)

The Ohio State University Medical Center provides their patients with a handout detailing the value of humor in pain management. By providing a distraction, humor shifts your focus away from the pain and onto whatever you're laughing at. It doesn't eliminate the pain, but it helps you deal with it more effectively. Humor reduces the prominent position pain plays in your day. *["As Dr. Smith, from 'Lost in Space' would say, 'Oh the pain! The pain'!"]*

What Humor Can Do for Your *Emotions*

Humor has a number of psychological benefits, too. First and foremost are the immediate benefits laughter offers: It makes you feel good. It lifts your mood and results in a more positive overall outlook. *["Sounds good to me!"]*

But that's not all. Humor can help you manage your diabetes by providing these other valuable emotional benefits:

Provides an Outlet for Anger

In my opinion, language was invented in order for people to communicate, whereas humor was invented in order for people to complain. Dealing with a chronic disease can trigger anger—and humor is a wonderful way to help process the negative emotions. Many comedians assert that their best material comes out of the times in their lives when they were angriest. (We did not ask Jon Stewart. We assume *his* best material comes out of Washington!) And while people will run like the building is on fire when a complainer approaches, humor can be a socially acceptable—even enjoyable—way for people to vent.

Part of having a chronic condition—any chronic condition—is that you're going to be frustrated, you're going to be angry, you're going to have moments when you are filled with rage. It's unrealistic to think that embracing humor as a coping strategy is going to eliminate those feelings.

But trying to ignore or stifle feelings of anger and frustration that come with diabetes just doesn't work. In fact, repressed anger and frustration can make your diabetes ever worse. Humor redirects anger, instead of avoiding or denying it. This redirection can defuse a lot of rage, bringing with it a sense of calm, relief and a fresh perspective. The underlying circumstances that made us angry still exist, but after we've laughed we're better prepared to address those circumstances.

"Laughter gives us distance.
It allows us to step back from an event,
deal with it and then move on."
~ Bob Newhart

It feels good to laugh at problems, if only for a moment. This doesn't mean closing our eyes to reality. Instead, laughter allows us to reframe the issue and look at it anew. Sometimes a change in perspective presents the information we need to move past the anger.

Reduces Stress

Humor is a powerful tool for stress reduction. People with diabetes tend to have high levels of stress, if for no other reason than the fact that managing diabetes is a full time job in and of itself. *["And it's a full time job that doesn't pay anything!"]* Add diabetes management to a day already filled with career and family obligations, and stress is the inevitable result.

Humor is recognized as a *healthy* coping mechanism. Sure eating, drinking and smoking to excess may feel good temporarily—but they can make you sicker, even kill you, in the long-run. Humor relieves anxiety and tension, provides a healthy escape from reality, and lightens heaviness related to those aspects of diabetes that really weigh you down.

A Time for Mirth, a Time to Mourn

Laughing can't cure everything. One of the things that is very real, yet seldom talked about, is the grieving aspect that comes with being diagnosed with diabetes. In the first place it's not at all uncommon (meaning—this happens to everyone!) for people who have just learned that "What's wrong with me?" isn't just the flu or being over-tired or a psychiatric breakdown, but is, instead, a disease that will be with them for the rest of their lives.

"I told the doctor that I've always been immature, but wasn't this stretching things a bit too far?" asked Jill Knox, who was 59 years old when she was diagnosed with Juvenile Diabetes. After a five-day stay in the hospital, Jill wasn't sure she was ready to go home on her own. "I was so afraid. I was nervous that I was going to overdose or underdose myself, and die during the night. It's a big responsibility. There are big consequences if you make a mistake."

You get no choice in the matter. If you recall (think back really, really hard here), at no time did someone take you to the side and say, "We're making a little trip down to Discount Dave's Disease Emporium—Where Debilitating Diseases Come Cheap!" You didn't get to say, "No, I'd rather have Parkinson's" or "Perhaps I'd look good in Depression." You're stuck with the diagnosis you've been given; you don't get to choose.

So we have a situation where we don't like the circumstances we're in, and we didn't get to make a choice about whether we want those circumstances in our lives. This is a pretty serious thing here, and it's sad. There will be times you'll want to mourn this loss. There's no need to feel ashamed, pressured, or silly about this. It's a natural part of the process. It happens to everyone.

It's also, believe-it-or-not, one of the best sources of humor in the world. I'd like to draw your attention to Rodney Dangerfield for a moment. Love him or hate him, you've got to respect the fact that he's built an entire career out of the fact that he gets, well, no respect. Getting no respect is not something Rodney chose, nor is it something he wanted. (At least not at first. Eventually it started working for him.) But he took that concept and used it to build a life of laughter. When we are done mourning, we can do the same.

Be aware that mourning isn't an all-or-nothing deal. It happens. Grief comes and goes; you're feeling fine one minute, and then something happens that throws you right back into a discouraged mood. It could be the baker running out of your favorite cookie; it could be the fact you have to think about your sugars when no one around you has to worry about anything; it could just be one of those days when you crash. The thing to do is to mourn when you need to and then let it go. Think of it as an exercise your psyche must go through periodically in order to keep in shape. It's necessary, but you don't have to stay in that mode all of the time.

And last but not least, Steve Wilson, founder of World Laughter Tour, had this to say: "Even if there were no evidence whatsoever that laughter changed a thing in your physiology—I want a life filled with laughter and humor. Laughter is its own reward, darn it. It feels good! Humor helps me see the world in better balance. Good natured laughter connects me to others, and that feels great. And, a life absent of laughter and humor is too dreadful to contemplate."

["Amen, brother!"]

What Humor Can Do for You *Socially*

Laugh and The World Laughs with You

One of the more subtle yet very devastating effects of a chronic condition is isolation. Diabetes can get in the way of relationships. From friends who 'mother' you in the hopes of preventing you from suddenly scarfing down an entire loaf of bread in a moment of madness, to co-workers who act as if you're contagious—there's a constant pressure on all of your relationships. And sometimes your relationships just can't stand the strain.

Humor is an effective way to combat social isolation. You can use humor to directly address some of the issues that crop up in your relationships. For example, if a friend wants to act like she's your mother, *treat* her like she's your mother and ask her for twenty bucks! *["I love this idea!"]*

> *"Laughter is the shortest distance*
> *between two people."*
> ~ Victor Borge

Humor has been found to strengthen existing relationships (which is good if you *like* the people you know!). Regular use of humor is thought to make us more attractive to other people, which can increase your social circle and your base of support (this is good news if you *don't* like the people you currently know).

Finally, the one thing you're absolutely certain to do as a diabetic is to be introduced to lots and lots of newly diagnosed diabetics. (It's true. The latest research indicates that most "persons-with-diabetes" [PWDs] are introduced to newly diagnosed PWDs a minimum of 38 times over the course of five years. That works out to roughly seven new people per year, or one every seven weeks or so. This of course assumes that humans will act in a regular, predictable pattern, and that doesn't always happen. Don't be surprised if you don't meet anyone with diabetes for four years and 364 days—and then meet 38 PWDs the very next day. Statistically, it has to happen to someone!) *["I had no idea that I was a PWD!"]*

These new diabetics tend to have lots of questions. Luckily, there are lots of people out there who can teach them about counting carbs and the wonders of exercise. *["Yeah, I rolled my eyes, too."]*

My suggestion is to let someone *else* handle that clinical and boring stuff. You can have some real fun instead by teaching the newbies about the little-appreciated value of *humor*. Share some of your favorite funny stories. Let's say you tell the tale of the hypoglycemic episode that woke you up in the middle of the night to rake leaves—in the middle of January! *["Who hasn't done **that**?!"]* You'll be doing more than making people laugh. You're sharing your own diabetic experiences, letting other people know that these things happen, and that they're survivable. There's a lot of comfort delivered with those chuckles. You'll be leading by example, and removing some of the fear the 'new guy' may be feeling. Let him know it's okay to laugh.

Levels the Playing Field

A little humor helps to break down awkward moments between people. It doesn't matter what race you are, what gender or what religion you are, or how much money you make (or don't make). If something's funny, people laugh.

Laughter reduces social hierarchies, making it easier for people from all different types of life circumstances to connect with each other. When we can laugh together, communication becomes easier. Whether it's a doctor/patient, boss/worker, parent/child, or some other relationship, when people are enjoying true mirthful laughter, they're on a level playing field.

Sarah is a longtime diabetic. She recently began seeing a new endocrinologist who was highly recommended but made her feel like she was a bother when she began asking questions. She says that when the doctor began falling into medicalese (a special language understood only by other doctors, sometimes used to discourage laymen from asking questions) that she told him a funny story about an airline security agent who was convinced that her insulin pump was some type of terrorist device. She and the doctor had a good laugh together, and after that she felt like he saw her as a person, not just "the 27 year-old T1 in exam room 2."

What Humor Can Do for Your *Communication*

Gets Your Message Across

One of the cool things about humor is that it helps convey information efficiently and effectively. Teachers, preachers, speakers, and politicians all agree; if you want to get someone *listening*, get them *laughing*. People enjoy laughing: When you've provided them with something humorous to enjoy, they're more likely to listen to the rest of what you have to say in the hopes that they'll get to laugh again.

Humor can serve as a safety net for difficult conversations. The ability to frame topics as potentially humorous material allows you to bring up serious subjects while "testing the waters" with your audience. If they respond well to the joke, it becomes easier to move the conversation on and address larger issues. Even humor that doesn't *work* can spark meaningful, much-needed conversations. Humor can open the door to important communication, whether it's with a doctor, nurse, family member or friend.

> *"Many a true word is spoken in jest."*
> ~ English proverb

On the other hand, there are times when humor can get it the way. If you have a serious concern, making jokes about it with your doctor or nurse may open the door for conversation. Then again, they may miss the cue entirely. It's not a good idea to use humor to evade a serious issue that may affect your health. You can't count on your medical team to be mind readers. If you have a concern, worry or question, ask them directly. Don't wait for them to bring the issue up. (And don't wait for the perfect straight line that will allow you launch into your comedy bit.)

Diffuses Difficult Situations

There are lots of ways to deal with difficult situations—but one that's frequently overlooked is humor. When moments get tense, whether it's a personal conflict or a professional issue, humor can diffuse anger, relieve tension, and level the playing field. Good communicators, like comics or politicians (or comics who become politicians; see: Al Franken) will have a list of savers or laugh lines that they can pull out when things unexpectedly go awry.

You never know when you're going need them, but if you can come up with your own saver lines, by being proactive you can give yourself more power and put yourself in control. Try this: Make a list of some of the things that might possibly go wrong and make up a list of answers that are humorous. Come up with at least ten and aim for twenty. (I'm covering my rear here, because the first few you come up with are going to be absolutely hysterical! *And* they're going to get you in so much trouble! I am not trying to cause you grief here.)

For example: The office nurse chastises you for putting on some weight since your last check-up.

Some possible responses to get you started:

"Why don't you weigh me in kilograms? It sounds so much better."

"I've put on weight? And all this time I thought I'd just gotten shorter."

"I'm wearing really heavy clothes today—mind if I take them off and weigh again naked?"

The last important point here: After using a humorous response, then address the problem at hand. The point isn't to get the other person laughing so hard that you can escape unnoticed (although that might come in handy for some really desperate situations). You're just trying to decrease the tension at hand so leveler heads can prevail.

"Nobody says you must laugh,
but a sense of humor can help you
overlook the unattractive,
tolerate the unpleasant,
cope with the unexpected,
and smile through the day."
~ Ann Landers

Chapter 3
Humor: the Good, the Bad, and the Ugly

Laughing *WITH* or Laughing *AT?*

The whole premise of this book is to convince you to use more humor in your life. That being said, some kinds of humor are healthier than others. When you stop and think about it, some kinds of humor make you feel really good. At the same time, there are other kinds of humor that can make you feel bad. *["Ah! I knew there was a catch!"]*

Take sarcasm for instance. Personally, I'm a real fan of sarcasm (like you can't tell?). And for sarcasm to work, you need to have a good connection with the person you're joking with. The root word of sarcasm actually means "to tear the flesh." *["Ouch!"]* And if you've ever been sniped with a sarcastic remark, you may feel like you were missing a bit of hide.

Humor comes in a number of flavors (and yet, it's sugar free!). There's *constructive* humor—the light, upbeat type of humor that builds people up. (A side benefit is that it builds *you* up, too!) And then there's *destructive* humor, which is a more negative type of humor, where we find the laughs at other people's expense. It is wise to avoid doing this.

People sometimes worry about their ability to tell the two types of humor apart. It's not as hard as you might think.

If you find yourself thinking, "I'm going to hell for laughing at this," it's likely negative humor. If you would feel ashamed if someone you respected—a parent, boss, friend—heard the joke, it's likely negative humor. If someone you didn't like told you the joke you were just telling, would you find yourself offended and incensed? Negative humor.

It's simply a matter of laughing *with* someone versus laughing *at* someone. It's always healthier to laugh *with* others than to laugh *at* them. Every once in awhile, your humor will fall into a gray zone—some might interpret it as positive, while others may find it offensive or off-putting. *["You mean I have to use my own judgement??"]*

One type of humor that usually works well is self-deprecating humor—making fun of yourself. No one will be offended, and it will actually show people that your self-esteem is strong enough to withstand being teased. Self-deprecating humor can actually increase other people's opinion of you!

A Word (or 872) About "Sick Humor"

One kind of humor that falls in the gray zone is "sick humor." Anyone who has to deal with an issue that is tragic, frightening, traumatic or unfair is a great candidate for sick humor (also known as dark humor, gallows humor, or black humor). That's why a lot of healthcare professionals love sick humor (tell a joke to an EMT about body fluids, death or dismemberment and watch him or her crack up). And seeing as how winning the Diabetes Lottery feels pretty unfair, you may be a real fan of sick humor, too. *["I love sick humor, but my spouse doesn't. So I have to watch 'Dumb & Dumber' in secret."]*

Note: Anyone who deals with traumatic situations is likely to count on some type of "sick humor" to help them keep their balance amid difficult situations. For example, soldiers, police and firefighters all have their own style of "sick humor" that actually helps them get by, and also bonds them to one another. It's a special brand of humor that is not meant for outsiders. And that's logical, because if you've never experienced what they have, you're not really a member of their "tribe."

Any kind of humor that makes you laugh, whether it's sick or not, is going to relieve your stress. It may not, however, do much for the stress of the people around you. Those who share your pain and experiences will "get it." Those that don't, won't.

Risky Business (and the B.E.T. Method)

Have you ever tried to be funny and put your foot in your mouth? On the other hand, have you ever put your foot in your mouth and you weren't even *trying* to be funny? There's almost always some degree of risk involved when you use humor. The purpose of our conversation is to push the cost/benefit ratio into the plus column. Here are some ways to take some of the risk out of the risky business of humor, and make your humor a safe B.E.T. (B stands for "Bond"; E stands for "Environment"; and T stands for "Timing."

$B = Bond$

The Bond represents those areas where you have a point of commonality with the people you're about to share your humor with. Where are you connected? Are they family? What are their ages? Are they work colleagues? Are they neighbors (close neighbors vs. casual neighbors)? High school pals? Drinking buddies? Do you have a close relationship with the listeners, or are you not so sure of what will make them laugh?

Use some common sense here. Consider the people you're with at the time. Are they the type of people who get offended very easily? Maybe you want to hold off on the humor. On the other hand, if someone starts the conversation off with her favorite joke, you're probably safe using some humor of your own.

The longer you've known the person and the better the relationship is with him or her, the safer your humor will be. If you've shared some gross-out humor with your best friend over the past 20 years, she's probably going to overlook the ickiness, not be offended, and will likely laugh heartily. However, if it's someone you've known for only a short time, or have only known casually, you may want to mentally edit some of your humor before sharing it with them.

$E = Environment$

Being aware of the environment also helps determine if humor is appropriate. There's a saying that, "There's a time and a place for everything," and environment is all about the place. For humor to be effective, you need your audience to be in a place where they're comfortable with humor. Some people don't joke in the workplace or in houses of worship, for example, but have no problem laughing it up in more casual settings. Not all types of humor work in all environments: The joke you tell while you're out at a club might not be the same joke you tell during a family gathering.

Anyone who hears your humor, sees your humor or experiences your humor is part of your audience, whether you meant for them to be or not. Maybe you're telling an off-color joke to your BFF at lunch but you tell it loud enough for the table behind you to hear—the family of four including two kids with big ears. Or maybe you're posting some inside humor on your Facebook page or on a blog site. That's fine as long as you're cool with the fact that some folks (including potential future bosses or dates) may see it even though it's not written with them in mind.

I've been in many hospitals in which the nurses stations or administrative cubicles display some Dilbert cartoons or some funny quotations. Here's the question: Will the displayed humor amuse or offend the patients or their visitors?

$T = Timing$

Timing is perhaps the most difficult element to master when using humor. Comedians spend countless hours trying to perfect their comic timing; some consider it a gift you either have or you don't. Luckily, you don't need Seinfeld-perfect comic precision; common sense will get you close enough.

The other thing to remember about humor is that it frequently comes from pain or discomfort. When do people find that kind of situation funny? *When they can emotionally detach from it.* Have you ever found yourself saying, "Someday I'm going to laugh about this"? Here's a suggestion: Try shortening the time frame. (It will take a little time, usually. At the peak of a crisis things usually aren't that funny...)

Some people can distance themselves immediately. They can laugh at their own mistakes—whether it's getting lost while driving somewhere, or saying something dumb in front of work colleagues.

But other people need more time to process their reactions and emotions. When some people get lost, they berate themselves harshly. And as long as they are emotionally attached to the painful event, they will not find it funny.

And there are those who will just *never* see the situation as funny. *["But where's the fun in that?"]*

> *"Someday we'll laugh about this."*
> ~ Richard Nixon to a White House aide

When to Use Humor

Sometimes it is difficult to tell whether humor is appropriate in a given situation. Many times, we're so worried about whether laughing is really the right thing to do at any particular moment, that we censor ourselves, stopping ourselves from using humor.

This is the "When in doubt, leave it out" approach. This is undoubtedly the safest option. Use it too often, however, and you may leave yourself unable to capitalize on some of the many benefits of humor.

It's also important to remember to refrain from using humor during moments of crisis, or when it's vitally important that communication be clearly understood. Humor works by distracting the attention, and there are times when distraction is a very bad idea.

Say you're blood sugar dropped and you got dizzy, then fell into the arms of a Matt-Damon-look-alike, and spilled your Starbucks-Grande-Decaf-Americano all over his nice khaki pants. You *could* go home and fall on your sword (or syringe); or you could wait a year before leaving the house again—*or* you could look for the humor in the situation and have a good laugh by saying something like, "I'm sorry sir, but I seem to have spilled my Starbucks-Grande-Decaf-Americano on your pants. If you take them off I'll have them dry cleaned and back to you within the hour."

Before using humor, do a quick check:
o   What's my *connection* with the audience?
o   Is this the right *setting* for this type of humor?
o   Is this the right *time* to use humor?

The Safest Form of Humor

When in doubt about what kind of humor to use with others, use self-effacing humor, or making fun of yourself. Sharing a funny story about yourself shows self-confidence and yet also shows vulnerability. People find this kind of humor totally non-threatening and may feel secure enough to share their own personal humor back with you.

With self-effacing humor, it's best to focus on the funny or dumb thing that you *did*, and not position *yourself* as being dumb. Using self-effacing humor requires self-confidence, and a strong sense of who you really are.

> *"I always wanted to be somebody, but*
> *I should have been more specific."*
> ~ Lily Tomlin

Remember this: You *are* somebody. Somebody who can be strong enough and confident enough to poke fun at yourself. Remember this, too: People who never use self-deprecating humor are not as confident and strong as they would like you to believe. In fact, they're scared.

That's a little tidbit to keep in mind while using humor. Self-deprecating humor—the bit where you laugh at yourself—is a strong and powerful technique to help deal with chronic conditions, not to mention everyday life. When you've left your testing kit inside again and you don't realize it until after you've locked yourself out of the house and missed the carpool to work, what can you do but laugh? The trick to self-deprecating humor is to make sure you focus on the things you *do*—and not the person you *are*.

"Laugh at your actions and not at who you are.
*It's safer to admit that you **made** a mistake than to admit*
*you **are** a mistake.*
~Terry Paulson, PhD

Seriously. The world does enough to tear us down. We don't have to do it to ourselves.

*"I realize that humor isn't for everyone
It's only for people who want to have fun,
enjoy life, and feel alive."*
~ Anne Wilson Slchaef

Chapter 4
You Want Me to Do
What?!

— or —

Taking Action

Now that you know the benefits of humor, let's talk about how to make humor a regular part of your diabetes management. The most difficult part of any chronic condition is seldom the condition itself, it's the *chronic* part. Managing diabetes day-in and day-out is a real challenge. In this section, we discuss humor strategies that will see you through the day-by-day nature of life with diabetes.

> *"The most wasted day of all is that in which we have not laughed."*
> ~ Nicolas Chamfort

I've listed over two dozen ways for you to incorporate humor into your self-care. This is to give you a range of options. Think of this as the Grand Buffet of Humor. Don't feel obligated to pile everything onto your plate. Humor is deeply personal. You'll benefit most if you choose and practice those techniques and strategies that resonate with you. Everyone has a personal comfort level with humor and will prefer some techniques over others.

I've divided the techniques into three primary categories: Manipulating Your *Environment*, Manipulating Your *Mindset*, and Setting the *Pace*.

Life is Like a Dogsled Team (Manipulating Your *Environment*)

Humorist Lewis Grizzard once wrote, "Life is like a dogsled team. If you're not the lead dog, the scenery never changes." It's up to you to take the lead in your own life. Don't assume someone else is going to step in from the sidelines and make your life more fun. You've got to take action.

Incorporating humor into your diabetes management means being proactive. There are simple steps you can take to cultivate the presence of humor in your life. Altering your physical surrounding can have a direct and dramatic influence on your mood. (That's why people go to the beautiful beaches of Hawaii for vacation: Simply *being* there can make you feel good!) In this section, I'll talk about the ways you can change your environment positively.

The Power of Play

Playful people are happier people. Happy people are healthier people. One of the best ways to introduce humor into your day and more efficiently manage your diabetes is to embrace the power of play.

Playing, having fun, using the imagination—once upon a time, these were our only jobs in the world. When we were kids, life was all about playing. Then, as the adult responsibilities began piling up, less and less time became available for playing. We've gotten too busy to have fun.

The *time* for play may have disappeared, but the

need for it has not. Today we need our imagination, our silliness, our make-believe and clever games just as much as we did when we were kids. Perhaps even more. Play is incredibly powerful—it lifts the spirit, rejuvenates and energizes, and adds a much needed element of joy to your day.

Play is powerful, and yet it is almost universally undervalued. Trust me, I've been paying attention (to children, to adults, to patients with many diseases, and to the medical and scientific journals). *["Well, I'm grateful that **someone** is doing all that. I'm too exhausted to do it all myself!"]*

Because children play, we consider play a childish thing. Yet nothing could be further from the truth. Play can transform the way we see the world. For example, there are contact lenses that change color in response to your sugar levels. Obviously, this is a great and easy way to monitor yourself without sticking your finger. *["That's mildly brilliant!"]*

But look for the play potential here! On the day that the office is gathering for the dreaded 'staff photo'—wear only one color-changing lens! *["Don't do this for your driver's license picture; the cops will never believe you!"]*

There's also tattoo ink that changes color with blood sugar levels. *["No way!"]* Most diabetic tattoo fans are getting discreet dots or subtle designs, but if you're a person who appreciates good ink and permanent play, what would be funnier than a tattoo that says "Life is Sweet!"? (If your future plans include doing a stint in prison, I totally understand if you opt for a different design. Perhaps a skeleton with a flaming test strip?)

Moving from the durable medical equipment arena, you can still play. If you want to incorporate more play into your life:

Create a Play List full of things that are fun for you! It can include games, playing with your kids or your dog (or your kids' dogs, or your dog's kids), skating, playing video games, etc. At least half the list should be low-cost or no-cost (unless you're both rich *and* diabetic, in which case go wild—and make sure your list includes, "Send large sums of money to my favorite author!").

When you're feeling down or it's been a really bad day, do at least one thing on your Play List. There is a method to the madness here. When you're most in need of play is when you're least able to think of something fun to do. You're feeling sick or tired or frustrated—nothing sounds like much fun. And sometimes you're feeling like gum on the bottom of a shoe because your cash flow is so slow.

So do not wait until you feel better to do these things! Do them when you're feeling bad, and I promise, you will feel better.

> *"What if the Hokey Pokey really*
> *is what it's all about?"*
> Bumper sticker

Because really, is it possible to have a bad time while dancing the Hokey Pokey?

Build Your D-Team

Surround yourself with funny people! You want to build a team of positive people who enjoy life, like to laugh, and know how to have a good time. I call this the D-Team, for the Delightful Team *["Not **every** D-word needs to be 'Diabetes'!"]*

This team has a critical role: To help you laugh

more. Laughter is contagious. You can certainly enjoy humor when you're alone—but you're more likely to laugh and have fun when you're with others.

Research indicates that we're up to 30 times more likely to laugh when we're with others than when we're alone. (Who did this research? Great question! It was Sophie Scott, a neuroscientist at University College London, along with her colleagues. Hey, I really don't just make-up this stuff, you know!) Our brains are wired to mimic the behavior we see exhibited by others; much the way you can acquire an accent when you travel far from home. When we see people laughing, we laugh too.

Capitalize on this tendency, and benefit from all the great things laughter can do for you, by creating and meeting with your D-Team on a regular basis. Taking in a funny movie, going to a comedy club, or simply getting together to hang out and have fun can all work.

At the same time, your D-Team can serve as support and reinforcement for your own humor campaign. From deflecting the "Diabetes Police" to always having six rolls of gauze on hand in case you hit a gusher while testing your sugar, the support of friends is critical.

"A true friend," Marie Z., an avid quilter, said, "is the one who points out that the moment after you've sliced your thumb open with a seam ripper is a great time to test!" (Marie Z. is a shy creature who doesn't want us to use her whole name, in case she becomes inundated by the fame and notoriety that comes from being quoted in a book like this. She *does* want you to know that she's a 43-year-old Type 2, who manages her diabetes well "except for major holidays, including Arbor Day, Flag Day, and Russell Stover's birthday.")

Think of your D-Team as external humor storage: They contain the funny that you may not have within you at a given moment. Call them on bad days or when you're having trouble coping. Let them lift you up.

Diabetes support groups can be great places to meet people who are navigating the same challenges you are. Give yourself time to find the right group. You want to find a group of likeminded people who share a similar outlook on life. Each group has its own personality and dynamic. You want to find one that is a good fit for you.

"It was so funny. The very first support group I'd gone to, and I mean the very first one, was going along fine until a man announced that the woman who normally ran the group wasn't there, and she wasn't going to be there, since she'd died in her sleep two days ago. And I'm sitting here thinking, 'This is going to lift me up? This is going to make me feel better?' Eventually I *did* find the right group of people, and it's made all of the difference—but I'll never forget that first experience!" said Jill Knox, on finding the right support group.

Being part of the D-team has benefits of its own. People who use humor regularly often find that other people learn to depend upon them to brighten the day. This can create a strong positive expectation, giving you an impetus to look for humor in order to pass it along—which cheers you up in the process!

Handcuff the "Diabetes Police"

One of the most amazing things about diabetes—and this is a symptom we haven't seen documented in the medical literature anywhere, yet—is how being diagnosed makes everyone around you an expert on your disease! It is truly astonishing how much "wisdom" the average layperson has about this complex disease, to say nothing of the compulsion they have to share this wisdom with you.

Well-intentioned or not, it's time to admit that there's something fundamentally annoying about having a relative stranger watching every bit of food you have on your plate and commenting that if you'd just skip all the white foods, you'd have no problems at all!

"People always say 'You don't look like a PWD'," says Kelly Kunik of Diabetesaliciousness (a blog dedicated to spreading information about diabetes through humor). "And I say, 'Yes, I *do*!' People can be such idiots about our disease."

There are four ways to stop the Diabetes Police in their tracks. (Actually there are *five*, if you count shouting "FREEZE!" at the top of your lungs. This will work, but only momentarily.) You'll want to pick the way that's the most appropriate for the situation you're in (think back to that whole B.E.T. [Bond, Environment, Timing] section we covered earlier).

The goal is to minimize the impact that the Diabetes Police have in your life, in a way that helps you preserve your energy and emotional resources. This is part of your self-care!

How to Handcuff the Diabetes Police!

Option One: *Educate Them*

Some people respond well to correction. Present the facts about your diabetes. For example, explain that, "No food is off limits—but some are more challenging than others, and I have to plan for them."

Option Two: *Walk Away*

You're not obligated to educate the world about diabetes. If someone is obnoxious, stubborn, or just not worth dealing with, simply walk away from the conversation.

Option Three: *Get Your Expert On*

Who has more diabetes knowledge than *you*? Let the Diabetes Police know you're thrilled to discover they're really an endocrinologist in disguise, and start bringing out all the multi-syllable medical terms while continuing the conversation, asking several incredibly complex questions along the way. (This method will not work on an inveterate 'truth-stretcher', who will rise to the occasion, making up answers as they go along. Use with caution—and on no account should you take their advice!)

Option Four: *Disarm Them with Humor*

"If it's sugar-free, I should be able to eat the whole thing!"

Humor disrupts the conversation, disarms the Diabetes Police's attempt to exert control over your life, helps you maintain personal autonomy and dignity, all while delivered with a smile and a chuckle. Many people with diabetes collect responses for use on the Diabetes Police; you may already have some!

Here are some of my favorites:

"Wow! Just eat healthy and exercise and my diabetes will go away? That's great! It's a shame it hasn't worked for your little weight problem there."

"Where were you when I was eating my salad?"

"280 is the new 120—haven't you heard?"

"You know, the Maori have found that eating eels stops people from getting diabetes! Have you had your eel today? Have

you? Why not? Waiter!" (Etiquette does demand that you be fully prepared to buy this person a serving of eel if it is available where you are. Yes, you'll be stuck with the bill . . . but boy will it be worth it!)

*"Remember when President Reagan defined ketchup as a vegetable? He did the same thing with **chocolate**!"*

*"And **your** blood sugar is...?"*

Be a Humor Collector

Some days, you're just not going to be able to find the funny on your own. That's the nature of dealing with a chronic condition. There are days when controlling your blood sugar is similar to herding cats (that is, next to impossible). You can do everything right and still have numbers that are sky high. There are days when everything hurts, no one understands you, and you are inexplicably without your flame thrower. (I would like to point out that I turned down a lucrative advertising opportunity from Flame Throwers R Us to represent them, because that's how I roll.)

But it's days like that when you really need a laugh. Stack the deck in your favor by building a humor collection that you can access whenever you need it.

What goes into a humor collection? Well, comedians, obviously. Although you'll need a pretty large house in which to keep them all. (It has been brought to my attention since writing this book that some comedians object to being kept in people's personal collections, preferring instead to have lives of their own. Go figure! So please make sure to ask your comedian if he or she has any plans before adding them to your collection!) That's merely a starting point, though.

A complete humor collection includes:

Funny Movies

Films, TV shows, and even the occasional sporting event can produce genuine laugh-out-loud moments. (Remember way back when we were talking about all the research regarding humor? Many of the studies observed people after they watched funny TV shows.) Build a collection of your favorites—and remember, they don't have to be funny to *everyone*, they just need to be funny to *you*! *["My TiVo is getting quite a workout—*

from 'I Love Lucy' to 'Late Night with David Letterman'!"]

YouTube is a treasure trove of funny videos. Create a favorites list of clips that make you laugh out loud for an instant pick-me-up.

Funny in Print

Build a library of books that make you laugh. Sometimes books are funny because of the content, while other books are funny simply because they exist. *Why Don't Penguins Feet Freeze?*, *Knitting with Dog Hair*, and *How to Hold an Alligator* are great examples—and you save money because you don't actually have to buy them; simply *knowing* about them makes you smile. (Yet another use for Amazon.com!)

Don't feel limited to books, by the way: Magazines and newspapers can be great sources of humor. *Reader's Digest* is known for its humorous anecdotes. Most magazines have some sort of humorous column and many major newspapers carry comic pages. (When are *The Wall Street Journal* and *The New York Times* going to get a sense of humor, and add a comic section?) And you don't have to be a kid to buy a comic book! (Just ask the 140,000 people who attend

Comic-Con every year—an annual event that every-one ought to experience at least *once* in their lives.)

Funny Art

There are all different kinds of art and some of it can be quite funny. The "StoryPeople" art of Brian Andreas can be humorous and profound, all at the same time. Keep your eyes open and you'll start to see everything from stamp-sized funnies (collect your Bart Simpson stamps) to yard-ornament-sized pieces of entertainment *["What lawn couldn't be improved with a collection of pink flamingos?!"]*

Better yet, create your own fun art! Participate in Diabetes Art Day. The brain child of Lee Ann Thill, blogger and art therapist, Diabetes Art Day is an ini-tiative to inspire the diabetes community to tell their stories through art (much of it funny, amusing, and incredibly creative!). And the very act of creating this art can boost your mood. Kelly Kunik (remember Diabetesaliciousness?) said that working on her art project for a mere five minutes put a smile on her face and lowered her stress level by *half*.

Toys

You don't need to have kids to have toys in your house or office. Get some toys of your own! Maybe it's a Slinky, or a Rubik's Cube, or a Koosh Ball, or the Pet Pancreas Talking Keychain (created by Theresa Garnero, a champion of diabetes education, and one funny, funny gal!). Maybe it's a water gun or a stress ball that you can squeeze the heck out of. It doesn't need to have a purpose other than to just bring a smile to your face when you play with it.

Cartoons

Cartoons, comics and other funny pictures can provide almost instant laughs and are yours for the clipping. But don't stop there! To get more mileage out of the cartoons, personalize them. Write in people's names or places of interest. Stick the cartoons on the fridge, tape them to your locker, mail them to a friend. Massage your creativity. White-Out the captions and write your own. *The New Yorker* magazine is well known for its cartoon caption contest. (Don't get the magazine? You can still participate online.)

You might think that cartoons specifically about diabetes would be hard to come by. But you'd be wrong! Diabetes expert and cartoonist Theresa

Garnero has a series of cartoons in her book, *DIABETease: A Lighter Look at The Serious Subject of Diabetes*. And Haidee Merritt will have you laughing out loud with her cartoon book, *One Lump or Two: Things That Suck About Being Diabetic*. Keep these on your shelf for easy access. Then take it another step: Try your hand at drawing some cartoons of your own. *["Even Charles Schulz had to start somewhere!"]*

Funny Audio

Humor on CD or MP3 is a great resource, especially when you're on the road. When traffic backs-up to a standstill and the guy behind you is laying on his horn, you can turn up the volume and laugh, instead of indulging in some free-form sign language. It's better for you and your blood pressure! (Do you remember Bill Cosby's classic and hilarious stories about "Noah" and "Fat Albert"? Do you remember that "Wild and Crazy Guy" Steve Martin? Do you remember George Carlin's "The Seven Words You Can Never Say on Television"? *["Oh my gosh, I remember laughing so hard that my sides hurt!"]*

FULL DISCLOSURE: If you like this book, you may want to get one or more of my CDs, too! Visit www.KarynBuxman.com. *["So, is Karyn being self-pro-motional, or merely helpful? You decide!"]*

Decorate for Laughs

Your living space (and by living space, I mean both your home *and* your workplace—after all, some of us spend more time at work than at home) has a huge impact on the way you view the world, yourself, and any place where the two interact. That's part of the premise behind Feng Shui (the other premise being that if you let them, people will pay you large amounts of money to tell you how to arrange their furniture).

The same theories can be used to introduce elements of humor into your life. Altering your living space to make you laugh is simpler than you might think.

Embrace funny pictures and posters. Small figurines and knickknacks on a bookshelf can trigger a smile; seek out those objects that make you giggle and place them around your home.

At work, you can use your decorating efforts to inspire even more humor. Collect pictures of your colleagues and their pets—and see if people can pick out the pairs that go together. (Some people really *do* look like their dogs. Be prepared. You'll never look at a Basset Hound the same way again.)

Decorate your testing supplies. A silly sticker stuck on the side of the test strip box can provoke a grin. Lori R. "bejeweled" her test strip holder with adhesive gems from a craft store. "I like my bling!" she said, "I have to see this thing twenty million times a day, so I should enjoy looking at it!" (Another shy soul, Lori R. is a 17-year-old with Type 1 diabetes. She's got a fashion sense only slightly less unique than Lady Gaga's.)

Embrace Technology

No, this isn't all about your pumps! Through technology, we're all more connected than we've ever been before. The internet, cell phones, social networking, you name it—the entire planet is no more than a click away. It's pretty amazing.

Why not harness this power to make you laugh? Start with your voicemail. Record a humorous message for all of your callers to hear. (You can do this with your personal voicemail and your professional voicemail. The professional voicemail can be a little tricky, so use your judgment. Not everyone wants to laugh when they call the funeral home, for example . . . so this might not be the best idea for morticians.) You'll be amazed at how many jokes you'll get in return (particularly if you're really subtle and say something like, "Leave your name, number, and favorite joke!"). You'll laugh when you listen—and you're sharing the joy.

Use RSS readers or news aggregator programs (like Google Reader) to collect all of your favorite funny blogs and websites into one convenient location. That way you can get a daily dose of funny without having to go looking for it: A real time saver! (Don't have favorite funny websites or blogs yet? Give yourself a gift and take an hour or two to explore the internet. Google "Diabetes + Humor + Blog" and you'll be amazed at what you'll find. Of course you don't have to limit your search to diabetes-related material, but it's a good starting point, and there's great value to be found in having an online community.)

There are numerous sites that will deliver the joke-of-the-day (or the cartoon-of-the-day, the cat-photo-and-funny-caption of the day, the funny-horoscopeof-the-day—you get the picture) directly to your cell phone. Sign up for one. That way you have a guarantee each and every day that there will be something to laugh about—and you don't even have to remember it, the phone will tell you. *["I think my iPhone has taken-over my brain!"]*

Our enjoyment of humor increases when we share it with others. We're social creatures, which is a huge part of the reason social networking has become so popular. Check-out Facebook, Twitter, and a gazillion other sites. *["Does my Facebook picture make me look fat?"]*

Use your social networks to share and solicit humor. Posting a joke to a wall takes but a minute, and seeing the responses gives you an added boost. (Even if they're just smiley faces!) Ask for jokes and links to funny material—people love to share humor!

Bring Humor to Your Doctor

When you have diabetes, part of your environment includes a variety of medical facilities. The doctor's office, the (hopefully rare) ER visit, the trips to the pharmacy . . . the list is endless, and is part of the reason why managing diabetes often feels like another full time job on top of the ones you already have!

Introducing some humor into the process makes it easier to deal with. Bear in mind that this is something *you're* going to have to initiate. Chances are your healthcare professionals won't crack a joke—until you do it first. Once you've demonstrated that you're open to and enjoy humor, they're much more likely to give you something to laugh about.

"People with diabetes are always talked *at*, not *to*," says Kelly Kunik, of Diabetesaliciousness. "Once you use humor, doctors and nurses and everyone start to talk *to* you." *["Hmmm . . . Humor actually makes a person more visible. 'Fascinating,' as Mr. Spock would say."]*

Knowing that humor is a tool both you and your healthcare providers can access makes some of the more difficult conversations easier. Almost everyone reading this will go through the dreaded "weight conversation" with their doctor. "My doctor was kind of aggravated that I didn't understand what he was saying about a new eating plan," Marie Z said. "I responded by telling him this joke:

A doctor is trying to get his patient, an overweight man with diabetes, to lose some weight.

"I want you to eat what you always do for two days, then skip a day, then repeat this for two weeks. When you come back, you should have lost five pounds."

A month later when the patient returns, he's TWENTY pounds lighter! The doctor is amazed. "Was it hard to follow my instructions?" he asks.

"The first two days were easy. But every THIRD day I thought I'd die," the man replied.

The doctor was puzzled. "From hunger?"

"No," the man replied, "From the skipping."

"And that joke seemed to get through to my doctor," Marie said. "He became less aggravated, and took the time to answer my questions more completely." (We in the biz of applied humor call this transforming "Ha-Ha" into "Ah-Ha!"—changing humor into insight.)

Of course, in an ideal world, we wouldn't need to motivate doctors and nurses into giving us the information we need, but it's a nice resource to have on hand.

A Note About Timing

Bringing humor into a medical setting is fine—much of the time. However, if you or someone nearby is in a crisis situation, humor can be inappropriate and distracting, and take the focus away from where it needs to be. Use your best judgment.

Party . . . Just Because

Give yourself reasons to be excited. There's enough serious stuff in life—but no one says you have to give up your sense of fun, excitement and humor!

Create events or festivities "just because." Theme days are a great idea (such as Beach Day, 70's Day, Country Western Day, etc.) where you focus on doing something fun that is tied to the theme. The Beach Day could include a Gidget movie marathon; a Country Western Day could include songs that never made the big time ("You're The Reason Our Kids Are So Ugly" or "Get Your Tongue Outta My Mouth 'Cause I'm Kissing You Goodbye" or "You Ain't Much Fun Since I Quit Drinking"); and we don't really want to know what you're going to wear to the office on 70's Day!

This doesn't have to be a great big deal to deliver great big results. Just try integrating the theme into your everyday activities: Bloggers could post about the theme, inviting readers to share their stories. You could dress in the appropriate attire. Dare to be a little bit silly, just for the joy of laughing and making others laugh.

Theme days offer the opportunity to have a gathering that isn't necessarily about food. This cuts the Diabetes Police off at the knees—unlike most of our holidays which are celebrated with the ABCs (Alcohol, Baked Goods and Chocolate) when it's *your* celebration, *you* can set the menu! (It would be, perhaps, cynical, to suggest a fantastically healthy menu containing no white food whatsoever. Everyone else should love it, since they recommend it so ardently to you!)

These ideas work best when you have buy-in from your family, friends, or co-workers. If you're in a supervisory capacity, encourage your entire team to get involved: This boosts morale as well as your own spirits.

Change the Scenery

Diabetes management is all about routine and regularity. You know when your sugar is up, you know when it's down; you can sometimes almost set your watch* by it. (*Watches: Archaic devices used by the author's generation to tell time. If you are confused by this reference, just substitute the word "cell phone" and you'll be close. But you can't place a call with your watch.) Taking our medication at the same time daily, setting up regular times to go to the gym and work out, the routine appointment with the doctor—it can become a rut before you know it.

That's why it is essential to shake up the day and introduce elements of spontaneity and delight into your day. For some folks, it's the daily routine of diabetes management that becomes a drag. These tasks everyday can wear on your soul. If that's the case, you'll want to change things up.

The easiest way to do this, of course, is to give your testing equipment to a nearby toddler, and tell the rugrat to put it somewhere safe for you. The sheer challenge of trying to find out where that may be, using only your approximation of toddler logic and acrobatic skills, can shake up your morning for hours at a time. (And don't try to take the easy way out and ask the toddler where your meter is. Not because it's not sporting, but because—honestly??—they're not going to remember!!)

If you're not quite that open to adventure (also known technically by the pros as "sane"), you can still introduce some elements of serendipity and surprise into your day. Commit to trying something fun and new each week: Read a new blog; go to a new restaurant, a new activity or class. Take a new route on your daily walk. Listen to a different style radio station than you usually do. Sleep on the opposite side of the bed than is your habit (you may want to give your partner the heads-up on your experiment, first!).

"Novelty is the parent of pleasure." (Robert South said this. I'm not sure who he is, but in case you wanted to know, there you go. William Thackeray, on the other hand, whom I *was* previously aware of, said, "Novelty has charms that our mind can hardly withstand," which is a good quote too.) Provide yourself with a regular diet of new experiences and you will find yourself having more fun!

If I Hadn't Believed It . . . (Manipulating Your *Mindset*)

There are lots of techniques to proactively add more humor into your life. We've talked about manipulating the things around you. Now let's take a look at manipulating what goes on *inside your head*. This is the ultimate goal, because once you are able to create a humorous state of mind, you have a totally portable skill set that will serve you anywhere at anytime.

Raise Your Awareness

Raising awareness means using humor as self-care, both by recognizing the funny side of life and by cultivating its role in your life. What's so funny about diabetes? There's a reason I titled this book with that curious phrase. It's a good question. Diabetes is a serious, life-altering disease. What's there to laugh about?

Diabetes, in and of itself, is not particularly funny. I've examined the medical literature from every angle, and there's simply not anything inherently humorous about it.

Living with diabetes, however, is another story—and that's really what we're talking about here, isn't it? Diabetes is just a *part* of your life, not the *entirety* of it. And, frankly, much of the rest of your life is probably pretty funny.

Sometimes that humor is dark. "How do you manage the stress of diabetes with everything else that goes on in your life?" a patient on a diabetes forum asked. Only a few moments elapsed before the first funny answer was posted. "Exercise and psychiatric drugs!" *["Obviously, they were kidding about the exercise part."]*

The first step in using humor to help manage your diabetes is to acknowledge that while the *disease* isn't particularly funny, there *is* a role that *laughter* can play in handling the challenges that come along with it. Dark humor, sarcastic humor, clever wordplay, slapstick comedy, good practical jokes, bubbly friends, puns that will make you groan, and everything in-between can help you feel better.

This might mean changing how you view your diabetes. We're often taught that certain topics are "Off Limits"—too serious, too delicate, too impolite, too personal, too important, too critical to laugh about. It's time to let that go, at least where it pertains to your health. Understanding the role that humor can play in diabetes management makes that easier, as does practice.

Don't worry—the practice is actually quite fun. We'll be getting to that next.

Seek to Find the Funny

You don't have to *be* funny in order to *see* funny— and seeing funny is one of the easiest ways to integrate humor into your life (admittedly, not as easy as a pump . . . but as of this moment, no one's created a humor pump yet).

> *"If I hadn't believed it, I wouldn't have seen it."*
> ~ Ashleigh Brilliant

The very first step in seeing funny is to assume that there's funny to be seen. If your worldview tells you, "There's nothing funny happening in my life," then you'll be right. On the other hand, if you believe that the world is an amusing place just waiting for you to discover it, then you'll be right, too.

Let yourself believe that the world is full of humor.

Just taking this simple step will place you light years ahead of those around you who are in too much of a hurry to take a moment to see and hear and experience the vast absurdity and delight going on all around us.

The search for funny is really changing the way you view the world around you. In a way, you're cultivating a deliberate mindset—a lens through which you view the world, opening yourself up to a funny interpretation of everyday sights, sounds, and events.

Look for funny signs. My personal current favorite is the Wendy's restaurant sign that reads:

"BEAT DIABETES
BUY 5 JR. FROSTYS FOR $1" . . .

. . . which is certainly an innovative approach to effective blood sugar control (not yet sanctioned by the American Diabetes Association)!

Newspapers, magazines, television—especially local news broadcasts—and websites produce tons of inadvertent bloopers that can provoke a smile.

Here are some actual newspaper headlines. *["And if they don't bring a smile to your face, well, you need more help than **this**—or **any!**—book can bring you."]*

"Kids Make Nutritious Snacks"

"Miners Refuse to Work After Death"

"Squad Helps Dog Bite Victim"

"Queen Mary Having Bottom Scraped"

"Something Went Wrong in Jet Crash, Experts Say"

Listen for the funny things people say. Kids, friends, celebrities, politicians—they're all rich resources of material. There are quote books and numerous websites devoted to the amazing things people say. For instance:

Actress Alicia Silverstone: "I think the film *Clueless* was very deep. I think it was deep in the way that it was very light. I think lightness has to come from a very deep place if it's true lightness." *["Huh?!"]*

President George Bush: "I have opinions of my own, strong opinions, but I don't always agree with them." *["I have the same problem."]*

Child to grandmother: "Why doesn't your skin fit your face?"

You don't have to make this stuff up! Challenge yourself to write down something funny each and every day. Knowing you need to record something—*anything*—can help you train yourself to recognize and appreciate the funny moments that are all around you. It works much the same way a food diary does. (This is actually a *lot* more fun than keeping a food diary. And it makes for much better reading after the fact. Not that it's hard to beat pages of "1/2 c. rice, brown. 1 chicken leg, overdone, tasteless, and greasy").

The items in your humor journal don't have to be magnificently funny, although sometimes they will be. For example, one morning at a busy grocery store, I watched a harried woman with an overflowing cart just crammed full of groceries cut to the head of the Express Lane—"10 Items Max." (Apparently 27 cans of cat food only counts as one item in some people's minds.) She was curt with the cashier, explaining that she was in a hurry.

The cashier, not missing a beat smiled sweetly and said, "No problem! Which ten items would you like to buy?"

One technique to remind you to look for the funny is to put a small dot with a marker, pen, makeup, etc. on your wrist (not melted chocolate!). Any time you notice it throughout the day, stop, look around, and take note of what's humorous around you right that minute.

Celebrate Achievements

Don't wait for people to step out from the wings and give you the recognition you deserve. Practice enthusiastic standing ovations for yourself.

Your blood sugar's been under 100 every day for a week? Whoop it up and celebrate! Give yourself three solid minutes of applause!

Made it through the holidays, working out the carbs so well you could have a piece of old school pecan pie and two candy canes? That calls for the Woo-Hoo Dance of Triumph!

Stopped the Diabetes Police cold in their tracks? Nothing will do but an NFL-style end-zone celebration, complete with spiking a football. This is particularly amusing if your run-in with the Diabetes Police happens at work. (But if you happen to actually *be* an NFL player, don't do this. The penalty fee will cost you a boatload of money.)

If we can be serious for a moment (we *can*, but only for a moment), let's take some time to examine why this works. Positive reinforcement, boiled down to its purest essence, is the concept that "The behavior that is rewarded is the behavior that is repeated." (This was stolen from my buddy Rick Segel, co-author of *Laugh and Get Rich*. Don't tell him!)

It doesn't matter, technically, *who* does the rewarding. What matters is that you get the recognition and appreciation for the positive things you do to manage your diabetes.

Pragmatically, no one on this planet is as aware of your triumphs and achievements as *you* are—not your partner, not your parents, not your health care provider, not your best friend. Nobody knows you as well as you do. You are the person most admirably positioned to provide this positive reinforcement.

Of course, once you start the celebration, there's nothing to stop your friends from joining in. Fun shared is fun amplified—the more the merrier! (When you become aware of your friend's triumphs and accomplishments, celebrate them! It makes *both* of you feel good and allows you to benefit from the healing aspects of humor even more.)

Give Yourself Permission to Laugh Alone

Humor is among the most intimate and personal of emotions. What makes us laugh is highly individual and unique. I've heard it said that senses of humor are like fingerprints: No two are alike. That's how I knew for sure this concept applied to people with diabetes: Careful examination of countless perpetually perforated fingertips has revealed a dazzling (and sore) display of individuality. And what's funny to you may not be funny to someone else. (You're laughing hysterically at something only to have one of your co-workers look at you disdainfully and say, "That's not funny.")

"I'd just been diagnosed," said Paul K. (a 58-year-old Type 2 diabetic who looks like a lumberjack, or a football player, or a Mack truck—you get the picture), "and I had started taking Glipizide. One of the side effects, for me, was this pineapple sort of scent that began coming out of me. I mean, it would radiate right through my pores!" He laughed. "Who would have thought a big guy like me would turn-out to be tooty-fruity?"

Paul used humor to deal with an unexpected side effect. It worked for him, but not for his wife. "She thought I wasn't taking the whole thing seriously," he explained. "But I was seriously following the doctor's orders. What else could I do but laugh about the rest?"

What happens when you're the only person laughing? Sometimes you just have to say, "You know, I'm my own best audience. And I just do this for my own amusement." Yes, humor can be used to entertain and lift the spirits of those around you, but it's also effective and appropriate to use humor to make *yourself* feel better.

Think of it as self-care. It's not hurting anyone, and it's benefiting you. If you stop and think about it, very little of your self-care actually requires buy-in or participation from other people. Do you have an audience every time you test? Do you take your meds on camera so everyone can enjoy the moment? Do you have a cheering squad every time you take the stairs instead of the elevator? (If you do, could you send them to me? I've somehow misplaced mine!) Don't worry if other people 'don't get it'—they don't have to for it to make you feel better.

Actively Embrace Humor as Part of Your Treatment Regime

If you can do only one thing to manage your diabetes well, that would be coordinating with your medical team and doing what you need to do to keep the situation under control (totally the lawyers talking here. Not that they're wrong, but talk about a bunch of kill-joys!). But you don't have to limit yourself to doing only *one* thing to manage your diabetes. You have the freedom to embrace a whole range of treatment options, and humor should totally be on the list.

A small warning for you: While I *do* advise you to become more conscious of your humor, don't over-analyze it. A curious phenomenon that those of us in the "humor industry" have noticed is that the more you analyze humor, the less funny it becomes.

*"Humor can be dissected as a frog can, but the thing
dies in the process and the innards are of interest
to only the pure scientist."*
~ E.B. White

Consciously choosing to make humor a part of your treatment plan sounds, ironically enough, like very serious business. Thinking about what makes you laugh from an analytical point of view isn't something most of us do on a recreational basis. It's all rather intimidating.

Intimidating, that is, until you realize the vast number of laughs that are derived from pictures of cute animals with witty captions (thank you, www.icanhascheezeburger.com), physical mishaps (America's Funniest Videos, anyone?), and the foibles of society's 'beautiful people'(this is the entire reason for *E! News'* existence.). This is not particularly sophisticated material here—nor does it have to be.

What we're talking about is the process of identifying what makes you laugh, and taking steps to make that a regular part of your life. Humor is essential. You want to have it in your routine, right along with testing your sugar, and your morning workout. Consider your time laughing and playing as much a part of your diabetes management as counting carbs and making sure you have testing supplies.

Who says you can't enjoy something that's good for you? Think about it: The next time you're lounging on the couch, watching your favorite comedy, you're actually doing something to manage your diabetes! (Of course, if your significant other suggests that you could also help manage your diabetes by getting off your butt and helping him or her clean the garage, that might be a good thing, too. Good luck holding him or her off with, "In a minute, honey. I just have to see the end of *Home Alone—Part 2!*")

What's nice about humor as a diabetes management tool is that you can use it anytime, anywhere, as you see fit. You don't need any equipment. It doesn't cost any money. Humor is there when you don't have the energy to do anything else; when every other coping strategy fails, humor remains. And it's totally portable!

Bring on the Bingo!

Living life with diabetes brings with it more than its fair share of attendant annoyance, aggravations, and things that make you roll your eyes. Shouldn't something good come out of all of this?

I think so. That's why I've created "Life With Diabetes Bingo." Voila, the LWD Bingo Card:

Life With Diabetes Bingo

TEST STRIP FOUND IN YOUR CLOTHING	TELL SOMEONE ABOUT THE NEGATIVE CARBS IN CHOCOLATE	BRAIN FOG	6 ROLLS OF LIFESAVERS IN YOUR BAG	BREATH SMELLS LIKE JUICY FRUIT GUM
EXCUSE YOURSELF FROM WORK TO CHECK BLOOD SUGAR	ENDOCRINOLOGIST ON SPEED DIAL	TESTING- HIT A GUSHER!	ACCUSED OF DRINKING. (NOPE! KETOACIDOSIS)	TEST STRIP FOUND IN ODD PLACE
REQUEST TO SHOW A NEW DIABETIC THE ROPES	"SHOULD YOU BE EATING THAT?"	FREE BINGO SPACE!	OUT OF FINGERS TO STICK	NOTHING YOU CAN EAT AT DINNER PARTY: ORDER HEALTHY & BILL THE HOST
NATURALLY SWEET	BLOOD SUGAR LOWER THAN IQ	BORROWING CARBS FROM TOMORROW	"JUST AVOID WHITE FOODS"	YOU JUST FORGOT. BLAME IT ON LOW SUGAR
DIABETES POLICE!	TESTING= BLOOD ON THE CLOTHES	HOMELAND SECURITY MISTAKES YOUR PUMP FOR A TERRORIST DEVICE	SICK OF PRICKS	PERSON WITH MULTIPLE PIERCINGS/ TATTOOS FREAKED OUT BY YOUR NEEDLES

As you see, each square is filled with one of those special aggravations that comes with diabetes. As each one happens, cross them out—until you complete BINGO with five squares in a line crossed off. (Four corners also counts and special bonus for the day you are able to Black Out the entire card!)

When this happens, treat yourself to a reward—something that you enjoy, that makes you feel better, something that makes you smile. It's a nice way to off-set all the negativity. (I'd say something here about karma, but I'm not going to. I get that way every now and zen.) *["Bad pun alert!"]*

Prop Yourself Up

Keep a humorous prop handy. Tuck a clown nose in your desk drawer, Groucho glasses in your glove-box, and a magic wand near the microwave. This comes in particularly handy when you're confronted with a surly teenager who's gotten off of his cell phone long enough to stare longingly into the refrigerator and share his first words in two days with you:

"There's never anything to eat around here!" This is the perfect time to use that magic wand to make him disappear. Magical moments mean family memories!

Having these items near at hand makes it easier for you to make other people laugh—which will very likely make you laugh, too. Really, it's pretty difficult not to laugh when you're talking to the nice State Trooper while wearing Groucho glasses. It changes the entire experience, for both parties. (It may change the experience, but it likely won't make the speeding ticket disappear. Come to think of it, it may be wiser to save the Groucho glasses for the drive-through restaurant!)

Having funny props around can bring a smile to your face too, simply by the virtue of their presence. Fran London, creator of The Laughing Buddha, says, "There's something very powerful about having a collection of tangible items that make you laugh." If knowing you have a rubber chicken in your filing cabinet (under P for Poultry; or C for Chicken; or L for Lunch;) gives you a giggle, put one in there. You might want to give the temp a head's-up though: It can be a little disconcerting to find yourself confronted with unexpected "rubber chicken jocularity" in the office.

The resulting phenomenon is known as a "Fowl Mood." *["Another bad pun alert!"]*

There are two types of props. *Universally* humorous props are those that make *everybody* (okay, *almost* everybody) laugh. You have here your pinwheel beanies, giant clown shoes, and oversized candy necklaces. (If you don't think oversized candy necklaces are funny, try wearing one to work. Try wearing it in front of the Diabetes Police. Be the first on your block to debunk the transdermal absorption of sugar myth! It's like performance art with Pez.) *Personal* props are those items you keep on hand because they make *you* laugh. These don't necessarily have to be funny to anyone else. (Not everyone appreciates the comedic genius of Bobble-Heads; and no one else needs to know why that picture of Elvis cracks you up.) Mix and match until you find the right balance for you.

Let the Music Move You

Music can soothe the savage beast. (Our lawyers insist that we remind you to avoid facing down lions and tigers and bears armed with nothing more than a

CD player and *Celine Dion's Greatest Hits.* Tigers in particular are known to be fond of Canadian songbirds, and this can negatively impact your expected lifespan. Be careful.) A powerful tool that can lift mood, elevate spirits, and positively impact your emotional state, music can be a tremendous asset in helping you manage your diabetes.

The trick of using music to regulate your mood is to find music that's personally relevant to you. That's actually a little easier for people with diabetes. Sometimes it seems like you can't turn on the radio without hearing something that brings your numbers to mind:

Pour Some Sugar On Me — Def Leppard
Brown Sugar — Rolling Stones
Sugar Sugar —The Archies
No Sugar Tonight — The Guess Who

(Do other songs bring your sugar to mind? Email your favorites to Karyn@WhatsSoFunnyAbout.com I'm trying to see if K-Tel will do a compilation album!)

When all else fails, fall back on old favorites. See if

you can recall the theme song to *The Beverly Hillbillies* or *Gilligan's Island.* Try out your favorite Christmas carols. ("Grandma Got Run Over By a Reindeer" works really well for this, particularly in July.)

Expand Your Definition of Intimacy

Yes, we're going to talk about *that.* (In an all-ages, family-friendly-type of language. Otherwise, I'd be able to charge a lot more for this book!) Diabetes can have a tremendous impact on one's sex life, for reasons both physical and emotional. This can be a problem, as the connections we have with our partner are a critically important part of our lives. In fact, some people argue that this is *the* most important part of life. (Personally, I'd put my local comedy club in first place, but you'll have to take this up with my husband, who has agreed to put up with my quirkiness.)

When problems occur, we have two options. The tried and true do-absolutely-nothing-about-it-hoping-the-problems-will-just-magically-resolve-of-their-own-accord strategy is very popular. It somehow persists despite the fact that it doesn't work at all.

The second option, which I talked about with Dr. Ed Dunkelblau, the Director of the Institute for Emotionally Intelligent Learning, involves using humor and rethinking your definition of intimacy.

For many people, the definition of intimacy and the definition of sex are one and the same. Expanding the definition of intimacy to include more than sexual intercourse will benefit every couple, not only those couples that include a diabetic. This means exploring different kinds of touch, closeness, and the conversations one has with one's partner.

"Intimacy can be defined as the exchange of vulnerabilities," Dr. Dunkelblau said. "Which means it's critically important that the humor you share be positive humor." Positive or constructive humor is laughing *with* someone, not *at* someone. Bear in mind that we all have a fear of being judged or rejected in intimate situations; it is essential that we don't poke fun nor use mean spirited sarcastic humor during these times. (And here's a tip for the ladies: When in bed, never, never, *never* point-and-laugh at the same time.)

"Anxiety is at the root of many difficulties," Dr. Dunkelblau explained. "Humor reduces that anxiety, which has obvious physical effects. It's not unheard of for couples to find that time together, sharing laughter, can then lead them back to a space without that anxiety, to a place that is more enjoyable."

It's important to remember that no one is alone in facing this challenge: There are now increasing numbers of resources available, with specific tips and techniques to enhance intimacy while managing a chronic condition. Explore what works for you, and don't forget the value a good laugh can add.

Here are some specific resources for you:

www.Diabetes.org

www.FrankTalk.org

www.InvisibleDisabilities.com

www.WebMD.com

["And don't forget to check-out Karyn's website www.WhatsSoFunnyAbout.com."]

Set the Tone for Conversations

If you manage the message, you'll manage the day. When someone asks you how you're doing, don't just answer, "Fine." Enthusiastically answer, *"Incredible!"* and watch the startled smiles appear.

One of the most draining aspects of managing diabetes (and pretty much any other chronic disease, including life itself, which has a 100% morbidity rate. This falls into the category of "If I didn't laugh I'd cry.")—is people's unwanted questions and advice. "Why can't someone ever just ask how I'm doing?" asks George T., a 66-year-old Type 2 diabetic. "Every conversation turns into an interrogation about my health."

Even if you've got good news to report, it doesn't take long to feel like diabetes dominates your conversation. This makes it difficult to maintain the positive, upbeat attitude we're aiming for. It clouds that lens we were talking about earlier, the one you use to find the humor in the world.

But you have control over the types of conversations you have and the messages you put out there. Answering *"Incredible!"* when someone asks how you're doing is a great way. You're "derailing" the conversation by providing someone with an answer they didn't expect—and the answer is lighthearted and upbeat, which is often a different tone than what is expected.

You can also take control of the message by limiting how many times you're going to explain your health situation on any given day. Make an agreement with those near and dear to you that unless you say otherwise, they can assume that all is well on the health front. After all, you don't inquire daily about their cholesterol levels, migraines, and that embarrassing boil on their butt. (If you have people who just won't get with the program, make a point of asking them intimate details about their health on a daily basis. Preferably in front of other people. When they protest, innocently say, "I'm just *concerned* about you . . .")

Don't minimize your condition when things are going badly, but on the other hand, don't dwell on the small stuff when things are actually going pretty well. You'll find you get more meaningful responses and concern when this type of conversation is limited—and more joy when the alternative is funny stuff!

Catastrophize It!

A fat, round, quivering drop of crimson blood splatters directly onto your white slacks, missing the test strip entirely. Now you have to jab yourself again—and you've got a stain that's going to look absolutely fabulous as you're about to go into a meeting with the boss.

Sound familiar? Sometimes it's the small stuff that makes us sweat; the miniature aggravations that throw us off our equilibrium. It's tempting to minimize the impact of the steady stream of seemingly small incidents that distress, dismay, and discombobulate *["Now THERE'S a funny word."]* us—until, that is, we remember that it just takes one more straw to break the camel's back, one last grain of sand to empty the hourglass, one additional drop of water to fill the cup to overflowing and send waves of negative emotions and wild behavior everywhere. We cannot ignore these small things. Individually, they aren't much, but collectively, they are everything.

The trick is to keep things in their proper perspective. One technique to stop the small moments from accumulating into an unmanageable mass is "Catastrophizing." (Sometimes the name of this technique causes confusion. Rest assured, it has absolutely nothing to do with contributing to the ranks of male sopranos.)

Catastrophizing is a game you play by yourself. When you're confronted with an issue that's relatively minor—the blood splattered slacks, for example—ask yourself, "How could this be worse?" Each answer should exaggerate the situation.

To wit: "Well, I could have hit such a blood gusher that turns my pants red (and that totally doesn't go with this top!)" Now that's ridiculous, but you want to take it even *further* from there. Perhaps the blood will start flooding your office and the entire building will be evacuated. From there, the streets start to resemble a scarlet Venetian canal; cars and trucks are washed away to be replaced with gondolas. Soon, someone will start knocking the skyscrapers sideways, in order to add a more European flair to the whole thing.

Ridiculous? Of course. But at some point, you're going to laugh (or at least smile). And you're going to remember that you're freaking out over a drop of blood on a pair of pants. And from there, you can move on.

Practice Humor Visualization

It's always best if you can surround yourself with people who make you feel great, who make you laugh and that enjoy your company, as well. But let's face it.

Sometimes you're stuck with a person who is driving you nuts. What's a person to do? Practice the art of Humor Visualization, or the art of playing with your comic mindset. No one is going to know just what pictures you've conjured up in your head—unless you're laughing so hard that you give it all away.

For instance, you love your job, but there's that guy in the next cubicle who has driven many a former employee to drink (White Out, that is!) with his annoying habits. The next time he begins ranting that the coffee is too cold, try picturing him tipping over bacwards in his chair—with his expesive tie drenched with coffee—along with his computer, which is shorting-out! *["Now THAT'S funny."]*

What would your CEO look like wearing a curly rainbow wig and a red rubber clown nose? Could you imagine the most annoying customer in the world doing a Lady Gaga impression? The possibilities are endless.

Take a Mental Trip

This is somewhat similar to the previous exercise, in that it involves picturing something amusing in your mind. But in *this* case, you're going to tap into fun and pleasant memories. We all have the classic stories we tell to family or friends when we get together and reminisce. About the time Aunt Clarice (5 feet tall and 5 feet wide) fell on her back in the snow and flailed like a turtle on its back, screaming for Uncle Carl to come flip her over (you had to be there). Or how your brother snuck the car out on the Fourth of July only to have a sack of fireworks in the back seat get set off by a stray bottle rocket that flew through an open window and eventually burned out the interior of the entire car after a dazzling display lasting over 20 minutes (true story—just ask my brother!).

The trick is to start purposefully collecting a repertoire of these stories and tapping into them. It wouldn't hurt to write down a list at first. Then periodically, take a moment to think back to these moments of mirth. Your body can't tell the difference between a *real* humorous event in the moment or an *imagined* event that is being recollected from the past. Both are going to do great things for your body chemistry.

Be Grateful

Gratitude is a powerful emotion. It's almost as powerful as humor, and when you combine the two, you can really benefit. So the trick is to find funny things about diabetes to be grateful for.

I realize this can be kind of tricky, so I'll give you a few of my favorites to get you started.

o   Conveniently timed lows can get you out of that exam you 'forgot' to study for.

o   Be able to tell anyone who is nervous about getting a flu shot or giving blood that he's a big baby. If he protests, tell him you were just needling them.

o   Enjoy the giddy feeling of living on the edge all of the time. "No . . . my middle name's not Danger, it's Diabetes . . . but it's almost the same!" (This line is lifted from the one James Bond movie no one ever saw.)

o   Your in-depth, up-close and personal relationship with diabetes allows you to speak with authority on the subject, and throw around polysyllabic words like they were confetti. (If, however, you're at a wedding, opt for the confetti. It's a rare bride indeed who enjoys her nuptials being showered with polysyllabic words.)

Laugh at Yourself

"You grow up the day you have your first real laugh—at yourself."
~ Ethel Barrymore

When all is said and done, you should take your diabetes seriously—it's serious stuff. But you can take *yourself* lightly. Learn to separate the two. *You are not your disease.* You are an amazing and amusing individual with a rich resource of life experiences. You just happen to have a pancreatic disease. *["Hey, some people get acne, and some get diabetes. Such is life."]*

Hopefully with the tools and information I've given you, you can put yourself and your life in their proper perspective. Laugh at your mistakes, your foibles, and your embarrassing moments, as well as your successes, your pleasures, and your joy-filled moments. Life really *is* too short to take it too seriously!

What are You Waiting For??
(Setting the *Pace*)

Start Your Day with Laughter

Mornings are hard. Is there anything harder than getting out of bed, especially if you know that's going to be followed by the morning trip to the gym? *["Especially when the route to the gym fails to include major attractions, like a Dunkin' Donuts or Starbucks!"]*

Behavioral researchers have found that the beginning of our day tends to set the tone for the remainder of that day. Dr. Robert Holden, of The Happiness Project, recommends that we ask ourselves, upon waking, "How happy do I choose to be today?"

You would think everyone would automatically say, "I choose to be super happy!" But that's not usually the case. Most of us have a 'range of happy' we're comfortable with: It takes exceptional events to make us happier than we normally are.

You can adjust those settings and expand your range of happy. One way to do this is to incorporate humor into your morning routine. Make sure you have something to laugh about in the morning.

This may reveal the underutilized value of humorous coffee mugs. (I received no financial support from the Humorous Coffee Mug Association to say this. However, if they would like to send me some cash as appreciation for this recognition, I'll be glad to accept it. You could also buy me off with a bunch of mugs—I'm clumsy, and could always use replacements.) Sign up for a joke-of-the-day email that's delivered first thing in the morning. Find a drive time radio show that makes you laugh. If you can't find anything amusing, fake it.

Experts have discovered that even *fake* laughter has benefits. (Not the least of which is that participating in laughter clubs and laughter yoga stands you a better than fair chance of showing up on local media, particularly during the slower periods of the news cycle.)

Several years ago, Charles Schaefer, a psychology professor at Fairleigh Dickinson University, conducted a study that demonstrated that even completely fake laughter can boost mood and overall well-being. In the study, participants were asked to laugh heartily for one full minute. Afterward, they reported feeling better, with a more positive outlook on life. The study was repeated with similar results, and has formed the basis of many laughter groups.

Laughter clubs can be found in many locations, particularly if you live near a large city. These can be a great resource, offering a chance to connect with other like-minded individuals. You can find out more by visiting www.WorldLaughterTour.com to find existing groups or to learn about forming your own laughter club.

Here are some laughter exercises you can try (and these will all work in the privacy of your own home, if you're more comfortable doing this where no one can see you!):

Flying Bird Laughter

Move around the room, flapping your arms like the wings of a bird, laughing all the while. Change the type of bird: Are you a slow moving albatross, gliding over the ocean, or a fast flying hungry eagle zooming to your next meal?

Electric Shock Laughter

Pretend you're getting an electric shock from everything you touch. Give a great big exaggerated response to every pretend shock: Jump up in the air, wave your arms, yell *"Aye Carumba!"* It won't take long before you're laughing like crazy!

Hula Hoop

Imagine a Hula Hoop around your hips. Get the hoop moving by swinging your hips in a circular direction—and laugh while you keep the hoop in motion.

Hearty Laughter

Laugh while raising both arms toward the sky with your head tilted a little bit backwards. Feel as if the laughter is coming from your heart. *["Frankly, at first, I thought this exercise was dumb. But I tried it—and now it's my favorite!"]*

Gradient Laughter

Start by smiling—then slowly begin to laugh with a gentle chuckle. Increase the intensity of the laugh until you've achieved a hearty laugh. Then gradually bring the laugh back down to a smile again. *["Is it normal to break into maniacal laughter, like 'Bwaa-ha-ha-ha!'?]*

Schedule a Humor Break

Make time for humor every day. This can be five minutes in the morning that you spend reading jokes online or the half hour you spend watching an episode of your favorite sitcom at the end of the day.

Anticipating fun can have nearly as many positive benefits as actually experiencing it. (There has been extensive research on this phenomenon, particularly by the Thursday-Sneak-Out-of-the-Office-and-Catch-a-Matinee-While-Everyone-Thinks-You're-at-a-Big-Important-Meeting Club.) For this reason, you'll want to load your calendar with fun events you're looking forward to. Movies, time with friends, an evening at a comedy club—don't view these things as indulgences; consider them a critical aspect of your diabetes management. *["Alas, not so critical that your insurance com-*

*pany will pay for them; good luck submitting **that** bill for reimbursement!"]*

Develop humorous traditions. If you know that the third weekend in March will always be your comedy movie marathon, where you gather with all of your friends and spend the weekend laughing, that weekend takes on a special significance and meaning to you. It also strengthens bonds and builds community: People who can never find a spare six seconds in their schedule tend to find the time to have a good time, particularly when they can plan for it in advance.

Planning for humor doesn't reduce the chances of spontaneous laughs happening throughout the day. If anything, giving yourself deliberate opportunities to recognize and enjoy humor actually prepares you to appreciate the funny moments in life when they crop up on their own. You're training yourself in a new way of viewing the world: *Look for the funny, and you will find it.*

On Your Mark, Get Set . . .

Go! What are you waiting for? There's no time like the present to get started and begin putting humor into your life starting right now! *When humor happens by chance you get some benefits—but when you begin using humor proactively you will create some amazing, life-changing results.*

Check back in and let me know how it's working for you. I want to hear your experiences. And I'm always looking for a good story or joke. *["Did you hear the one about...?"]*

*"Warning: Humor may be
hazardous to your illness."*
~ Ellie Katz

Chapter 5
The Last Laugh

So here we are, at the end of the book. I hope you enjoyed reading this as much as I enjoyed writing it (which was a lot!). It's better than working out at the gym, anyway... right? And packed with nearly as many benefits!

Adding humor to your diabetes management kit is painless and should be a lot of fun. Remember that the benefits of humor increase when they're shared— and besides, laughing with someone else is fun in and of itself!

Take time everyday to treat yourself well. You test every day, you watch your carbs every day (okay, every day that is *not* Halloween), you exercise every day— *["Really??"]*—all in the name of diabetes management. It's time to add *one* more element: *Enjoy humor every day.*

Laugh often, laugh deeply, laugh with others, and laugh alone. Laugh in the morning and laugh in the evening. Laugh knowing that you're reducing stress, helping your health, and most importantly of all, that you're having fun.

Humor is as crucial as insulin, as critical as counting carbs, and as joyful as discovering a sugar free version of your favorite childhood treat.

And here's one last joke, just to leave you laughing:

The owner of a music shop was just about to close his doors after a long day, when two very excited diabetics, George and Scott, came running through the door.

"Wow, is that sign for real?" Scott demanded.

"What sign?" the store owner asked.

"The one in the front window!" George said. "Is that true?"

"Well, of course," the music shop owner said. "That's what we do here."

"Then we'll take two!" the men exclaim, very excited. "One for each of us! Right now!"

"What?" the store owner asked, completely confused. "What do you want?"

"A functional pancreas!" Scott exclaimed.

"But this is a music store!" the shop owner said.

A look of confusion falls on everyone's face.

George sheepishly replied, "But the sign says "Organs for Sale!"

"The body heals with play,
The mind heals with laughter,
The spirit heals with joy."

~ A proverb

About the Author
Karyn Buxman, RN, MSN, CSP, CPAE

Meet nurse, speaker, author, publisher, and internationally recognized expert in applied and therapeutic humor, Karyn Buxman, RN, MSN, CSP, CPAE. She shows people how to harness humor and leverage laughter to reap the physical, psychological, social, communicative and even spiritual benefits.

Through her 25 years of research and experience, Karyn has determined that humor and its powerful effects help individuals live more positive, resilient, and healthier lives. "Humor by chance can be beneficial, but humor by choice creates amazing, life-changing results."

Her clients range from the Mayo Clinic to the Million Dollar Round Table and they hire Karyn to entertain, educate and inspire their audiences over and over again.

Karyn holds a distinguished position in the world of speaking. She has earned the National Speakers Association's (NSA) Certified Speaking Professional (CSP) designation, held by less than 7% of professional speakers, and is one of only 35 women in the world awarded admission into the NSA Speaker Hall of Fame (CPAE). She's received the Lifetime Achievement Award from the Association for Applied & Therapeutic Humor and is past president of this international organization. She serves on the advisory board of the Invisible Disabilities Association, as well as World Laughter Tour, and NurseTogether.com. She is a frequent media guest, has appeared in numerous magazines, blogs and professional journals, and is the publisher of *The Journal of Nursing Jocularity*.

Karyn is serious about humor!

Recommended Resources

(Online resources that can deepen your understanding of applied and therapeutic humor, and also about diabetes.)

Association for Applied and Therapeutic Humor, www.aath.org

This non-profit organization serves as the community for professionals who study, practice and promote healthy humor. Services include ezine, teleconferences, annual conference, CEs, and graduate credit available through the Humor Academy.

American Diabetic Association, www.Diabetes.org

The official site for the American Diabetes Association providing articles, resources, news, research and much more.

Comic-Con, www.Comic-Con.org

An annual gathering of 140,000 fans of popular culture, including movie fans, sci-fi fans, Star Wars aficionados, super hero lovers, and comic book fans.

DiabetesMine, www.DiabetesMine.com
This site was created by and for patients as a
"diabetes newspaper with a personal twist."

Theresa Garnero, www.TGarnero.com
Author of *DIABETease* and creator of the Talking Pet
Pancreas. Check out her cartoons and products here.

HUMORProject, www.HumorProject.com
Helping people improve their lives through the positive power of humor and creativity. Resources, articles,
and an annual conference.

Invisible Disabilities Association
www.InvisibleDisabilities.org
A non-profit organization providing education,
encouragement and community to anyone who is
touched by an invisible disability (whether directly or
though a loved one). They're raising awareness and
helping decrease the stigma of having an invisible disability.

Kelly Kunik,
www.Diabetesaliciousness.blogspot.com
Diabetes advocate, writer, humorist and expert at living life with diabetes. Bookmark her blog if you want to be informed, entertained and inspired.

Laughter Yoga, www.LaughterYoga.com
Founded by Dr. Madan Kataria, Laughter Yoga combines unconditional laughter with yogic breathing (Pranayama). Exercises, events, and information available.

Haidee Merritt, www.HaideeMerritt.com
Publisher, illustrator, T1, realist. Order her book, *One Lump or Two: Things That Suck About Being Diabetic.*

Lee Ann Thill,
www.TheButterCompartment.com/page_id+555
3 and **www.DiabetesArtDay.com**
Founder of Diabetes Art Day, Lee Ann encourages people with diabetes and their loved ones to utilize art as a way of communicating their experience with diabetes, connecting with others, raising awareness, and promoting insight and positive coping skills.

The New Yorker **Cartoon Caption Contest**
www.newyorker.com/humor/caption
A weekly contest where anyone can submit captions to a cartoon provided by *The New Yorker*. The winners' captions appear in the magazine. No cash prizes, but it's great for bragging rights!

StoryPeople, www.StoryPeople.com
Illustrations with funny and/or insightful thoughts, by artist Brian Andreas.

What's So Funny About . . .?
swww.WhatsSoFunnyAbout.com
Ongoing information on applied and therapeutic humor for chronic illnesses, from Karyn Buxman, RN.

www.WebMD.com. Great articles and resources.

World Laughter Tour, www.WorldLaughterTour.com
Founded by Steve Wilson and Karyn Buxman to support, promote, and act as a clearinghouse for the global laughter movement, with the mission of bringing events to every continent that promotes health and peace through laughter. Articles, exercises, events and news.

Appendix

(Scientific and medical research published in
official journals that back-up the claims made about
applied humor in this book.)

Chapter 1 Bibliography

2011 National Diabetes Fact Sheet, Centers for
Disease Control and Prevention
http://www.cdc.gov/diabetes/pubs/factsheet11.htm
?utm_source=WWW&utm_medium=ContentPage&
utm_content=CDCFactsheet&utm_campaign=CON

Amen, D. (2005) Making a good brain great. New
York: Three Rivers Press.

Cigolie, C., Lee, P., Langa, K., Lee, Y., Tian, Z., and
Blaum, C. (2011). Geriatric conditions develop in
middle-aged adults with diabetes. Journal of General
Internal Medicine, 26(3) 272-279.
http://www.springerlink.com/content/8031w211q82
qn067

Diabetes soaring among American adults. HealthDay, (2011). http://consumer.healthday.com/Article.asp? AID=648552

Diabetes Statistics, American Diabetes Association, http://www.diabetes.org/diabetes-basics/diabetes-statistics/

Gordon, S. (April, 2011). Add cancer to health risks of diabetes: Study, HealthDay. http://health.usnews.com/health-news/diet-fitness/diabetes/articles/2011/04/03/add-cancer-to-health-risks-of--diabetes-study

Li, C.; Balluz, L.; Ford, E.; Okoro, C.; Tsai, J, and Zhao, G. (2011). Association between diagnosed diabetes and self-reported cancer among U.S. adults, Diabetes Care. http://care.diabetesjournals.org/content/34/6/1365

Chapter 2 Bibliography

Berk, L.S. & Tan, S. (2006). [beta]-Endorphins and HGH increase are associated with both the anticipation and experience of mirthful laughter. The FASEB Journal, 20, A382.

Berk, L.; Tan, S.; Fry, W.; Napier, B.; Lee, J.; Hubbard, R.; Lewis, J.; & Eby, W. (1989). Neuroendocrine and stress hormone changes during mirthful laughter. American Journal of Medical Science. 298(6), 390-396.

Berk, L.; Tan, L.; & Tan, S. (2009). Mirthful laughter, as an adjunct therapy in diabetic care, increases HDL cholesterol and attenuates catecholamines, inflammatory cytokines, C-RP, and myocardial infarction occurrence. The FASEB Journal, 22, 1226.2.

Buxman, K. (1990). The professional nurse's role in developing a humor room in a health care setting. Masters Thesis, University of Missouri, Columbia.

Goldstein, J. (1987). Therapeutic effects of laughter. In W.F. Fry & W.A. Salameh (Eds.), Handbook of humor and psychotherapy. Sarasota, FL: Professional Resource Exchange.

Hayashi, K.; Hayahsi, T.; Iwanaga, S.; Kawai, K.; Ishii, H.; Shoji, S. & Murikami, K. (2003). Laughter lowered the increase in post-prandial blood glucose. Diabetes Care, 26 (5), 1651-1652.

Hayashi, T,; Urayma, O.; Kawai, K.; Hayashi, K.; Iwanaga, S.; Ohta, M.; Saito, T.; & Murakami, K. (2006). Laughter regulates gene expression in patients with Type 2 diabetes. Psychotherapy & Psychosomatics, 75(1), 62-65.

Hayashi, T. & Murakami, K. (2009). The effects of laughter on post-prandial glucose levels and gene expression in type 2 diabetic patients. Life Science, May 19.

Joel Goodman, EdD, founder of HUMORProject, 1989, presentation, Power of Laughter and Play annual conference, Tampa FL.

Lee Berk, PhD; Earl Henslin, PsyD., MFT, BCETS; Steve Sultanoff PhD; & Kathleen Passanisi, PT, CSP, CPAE; April 8, 2011 presentation, "Science Fiction, Science Fact, or What We Just Want to Be True," Association for Applied and Therapeutic annual conference, Anaheim CA.

McGhee, P. (2010). <u>Humor. The Lighter Path to Resilience and Health</u>. Bloomington, IN: AuthorHouse

Robinson, V. (1991). <u>Humor and the health professions</u>. Second Edition. Thorofare: Slack Publications.

Saturday Night Live, Season 3, episode 18, Theodoric of York Medieval Barber
<u>http://www.hulu.com/watch/3529/saturday-night-live-theodoric-of-york</u>

Sue McLaughlin, RD, certified diabetes educator, American Diabetes Association, The Nebraska Medical Center, Omaha; April 17, 2009, presentation, American Physiological Society annual meeting, New Orleans.

Stanley Tan, MD, MPH, MS, PhD, DTM&H, FACE, FCCP; April 9, 2011 presentation, "Laughter Is The Best Medicine, Scientific Evidences," The Association for Applied & Therapeutic Humor annual conference, Anaheim CA.

Chapter 3 Bibliography

Robinson, V. (1991). <u>Humor and the health professions</u>. Second Edition. Thorofare: Slack Publications.

Gross, T., Buxman, K., & Ayers, G. (2009). <u>The service prescription</u>. Healthcare the way it was meant to be. La Jolla CA: LaMoine Press.

Chapter 4 Bibliography

The glucose-monitoring tattoo: A novel nanosensor could be useful for skin-based glucose screening. (1-26-2009). <u>Technology review</u>. http://www.technologyreview.com/biomedicine/22014/

Color-change lenses check blood sugar. ABC News. (April 2011). http://abcnews.go.com/Technology/FutureTech/story?id=97664&page=1

Garnero, T. (2003). <u>DIABETease: A lighter look at the serious subject of diabetes</u>.

Grizzard, L. (2001). The wit and wisdom of Lewis Grizzard: Life is like a dogsled team. Athens GA: Longstreet Press.

Kataria, M. (1999). Laugh for no reason. Andheri, Mubai: Madhuri International.

Kunik, K. (2011). http://www.Diabetesaliciousness.blogspot.com

Merritt, H. (2009). One lump or two: Things that suck about being diabetic.

Segel, R. & LaCroix, D. (2000). Laugh and get rich. Burlington, MA: Specific House.

Simonton, C., & Henson, R. (1992). The healing journey. New York: Bantam.

The neuroscience of laughter. All things science. http://www.dailymotion.com/video/xhqany_the-neuroscience-of-laughter_tech

Wilson, S. (2011). http://www.Worldlaughtertour.com/sections/news/articles.asp

Index

"Humor by chance can be beneficial,
but humor by choice
creates amazing, life-changing results."
~ Karyn Buxman